# SURVIVING DEPENDENCE:
# VOICES OF
# AFRICAN AMERICAN ELDERS

### Mary M. Ball
*Georgia Division of Aging Services*

### and

### Frank J. Whittington
*Georgia State University*

### Jon Hendricks, Series Editor

### Society and Aging

Baywood Publishing Company, Inc.
Amityville, New York

Library of Congress Catalog Number: 95-7707
ISBN: 0-89503-125-6 (Cloth)
ISBN: 0-89503-126-4 (Paper)


**Library of Congress Cataloging-in-Publication Data**

Ball, Mary M.
    Surviving dependence : voices of African American elders / Mary M.
    Ball and Frank J. Whittington.
        p.    cm. - - (Society and aging)
    Includes bibliographical references and indexes.
    ISBN 0-89503-125-6. - - ISBN 0-89503-126-4 (pbk.)
    1. Afro-American aged- -Home care- -Case studies.  2. Old age-
    -United States- -Case studies.  3. Afro-American aged- -Long-term
    care- -Case studies.  I. Whittington, Frank J.  II. Title.
    III. Series.
    HV1461.B346  1995
    366.6'089'9673- -dc20                                    95-7707
                                                             CIP

# Dedication

To the magnificent seven

Mrs. Finch
Mrs. Little
Mrs. Oliver
Rev. Scott
Mrs. Starr
Mrs. Washington
Ms. Worth

Their spirit was our inspiration,
their words our reward.


To my family,
Turner, Eleanor, Caroline, Conner, and Steve
and to the memory of D. Scott Enright
—MB


To my parents,
Frank and Allee Whittington
my teachers about how to live and how to age
—FW

# Preface

The late summer sun was challenging our building's air conditioning, and I was fretting over a syllabus. A new graduate student appeared at the door to get acquainted and gauge her prospects in the new environment of doctoral study in sociology. She was older than usual but no older than some others I had taught and certainly seemed no older than I. She was soft-spoken—as are many southern women her age—but not shy. She seemed to possess both the uncertainty appropriate to launching a new career in mid-life and a degree of self-confidence, probably conferred by her two master's degrees, a full resumé of volunteer leadership and service, and years of childrearing experience. Neither of us suspected at that first meeting that we would become research partners as well as friends and colleagues.

This book is the result of our collaboration. To Mary it is the real culmination of her doctoral research and an affirmation of her commitment to understanding the seven older persons depicted here. To me it represents the best kind of mentor-student relationship, the kind every teacher hopes for. Of course, we all want to prepare our students for productive, independent careers. But if, during the course of the training, the student also can produce truly valuable new knowledge, the best of outcomes has been realized. During our collaboration, which has spanned Mary's five years of graduate study and the three additional years that were required to transform her dissertation into a publishable manuscript, both of these goals have been accomplished.

Mary was well-suited to the kind of research she wanted to do. In fact, she was meant to do it. Much of her training and earlier experiences had readied her for ethnographic field work among the poor and sick of the black community. Her graduate training in anthropology, gerontology, and qualitative methods and her twenty years' experience as a volunteer in a low-income community center in an inner-city black neighborhood all prepared her to enter, observe, and understand the lives of her study participants.

My role throughout the dissertation work was entirely that of director and mentor. I provided connections to the literature, judgments about theoretical and methodological problems, and advice on matters of organization and interpretation of the data. Later, as we worked on the project, we became colleagues, each with a particular set of abilities and insights. Mary knew intimately the participants, their community, and the data she had collected. She also had a greater understanding of ethnographic methods and their special advantages and drawbacks. My knowledge of the fields of aging and long-term care helped us establish a better context and refine the analysis, and my editorial experience was useful as we reorganized and streamlined the manuscript.

All collaborative work requires consideration and patience, and ours was no exception. Through my two years at the National Institute on Aging, a new job for Mary, and the marriage of her eldest daughter, our progress occasionally faltered, though never our resolve. Our experience as colleagues was both rewarding and revealing: both of us learned as much about ourselves as about how poor, elderly African Americans experience illness and home care. Although writing a book is often a long, fearful, and tedious process, our particular frustrations never seemed as numerous as our fascinations. And both clearly are evident in the pages that follow. Our aim is that readers will be as impressed, as entertained, and as respectful as we have been with the wisdom and wit, the determination and dignity of the seven elders from whom we were privileged to learn.

*Frank Whittington*

# Acknowledgments

Many people contributed to this project. Above all, we are indebted to the seven participants who welcomed us into their lives and whose words are the soul of this book. We are very grateful to the agency that administers the Community Care Services Program for providing entree to the study participants. We especially thank the case managers for introducing us to their clients and providing valuable information. Appreciation and respect also are due our participants' caregivers—both paid and unpaid—who welcomed a researcher's interest and questions.

Our colleagues and friends in the Sociology Department at Georgia State, Paula Dressel and Ralph LaRossa, have our deepest gratitude. By reading early drafts and giving us excellent advice on many topics, they were instrumental in the success of this effort. We acknowledge also our debt to our colleague, Scott Enright, whose commitment to teaching and using qualitative methods inspired this project. Our appreciation of his dynamic leadership was only sharpened by his loss in March, 1994.

Editors, someone has said, are a necessary evil. Ours at Baywood, Joe Hendricks, was certainly necessary to the successful completion of this book, but never evil. His guidance was as gentle as it was insightful and beneficial. We appreciate everything he did to bring this book into print.

We are deeply grateful to Turner Ball, Caroline Ball, B. J. Freeman, Joy Lobenstine, and Catherine Hennessy for their insightful comments on the manuscript. We appreciate also the diligence and care of Lona Choi whose research assistance supported and advanced our work.

Finally, we acknowledge the encouragement and support provided throughout this project by our families and friends—Conner Ball, Eleanor Ball, Steve Sencer, Frank Whittington, Allee Whittington, Kay Boykin, Jill Waldman, Mark Whittington, Tim Whittington, Eleathia Brown, Elizabeth Coleman, Lenore Conroy, Willard Pate, Gay Allen, and Chris Rosenbloom.

*Mary Ball and*
*Frank Whittington*

# Table of Contents

# Introduction

Mary M. Ball

*Oh, I didn't know it was going to be so hard. I know if you get older, you're gonna hurt. Just to depend on other people, that's the hardest part.*

Sally Finch

Being African American and poor helped ready Sally Finch for the battle of old age. Growing up during the Depression, she learned early how to work hard and how to do without. But this history of struggle has exacted its toll on her health and contributed to the dependence she so woefully laments. Like many Americans who live to see old age, she has multiple disabling chronic conditions. Being black and poor only hastened her fate and made it more certain.

Mrs. Finch is one of seven African American elders who shared of themselves and their lives, and this book tells their stories—stories of being old, black, poor, and no longer able to manage alone. In these tales we see what it means to live with dependency while trying to maintain important roles, relationships, and patterns of everyday living shaped by lifetimes of experience. We observe the quest for independence and the fight to have even simple needs met, and we learn how people adjust to disease, disability, and dependency and how they relate to those who care for them—both their informal caregivers and those who represent the public bureaucracy.

## RACE, POVERTY, AND HEALTH

The social characteristics of these seven elders leave them in a particularly vulnerable group. Evidence is clear that poor people do not live as long as the non-poor and that they suffer disproportionately from major diseases [1]. This relationship between poverty and health is affected also by other variables, such as gender, age, race, and

1

marital status. The oldest old are the poorest, and the youngest old, the most economically secure [2, 3]. Older women have a higher poverty rate than men (16% vs. 9%), and about one-third (33%) of elderly blacks are poor—a rate three times that of elderly whites (11%) [4]. At the intersection of race and gender, data show that white men are better off than white women, white women fare better than black men, and black women are the poorest group [5]. In addition, being unmarried also is strongly associated with poverty, and because they tend to outlive their husbands, women are more likely to be unmarried than men [2].

The relationship between race and health, like that between poverty and health, is complicated by other demographic variables. The predominance of women among elderly blacks and their greater likelihood than white women of being unmarried and poor all contribute to the differences in health status of blacks and whites [6, 7]. Although prevalence rates of the most common chronic conditions are similar for blacks and whites [6], available data on limitations in daily activities indicate that older blacks have a higher level of functional dependency than whites, particularly among poor old women [8-10].

## CARE NEEDS, CAREGIVERS, AND CARE COSTS

As we shall see, the needs of these seven African American elders reflect all too well the growing long-term care needs of the oldest sector of the American population, a now familiar story. Despite comparisons of data from the 1984 and 1989 Long Term Care Surveys that suggest declines in chronic disability prevalence in the U.S. elderly population, absolute increases in long-term care needs still are predicted [3]. Trends indicate that one in four persons eventually will need some type of long-term care [11]. Age is the principal determinant of need for these services. According to the U.S. Senate Special Committee on Aging, in 1988 about seven million people needed assistance taking care of themselves. By the year 2020, it is estimated that over twelve million will need long-term care [12].

While only 5 percent of the elderly population are in a nursing home at any time, the percentage is dramatically higher among the oldest old—36 percent for persons ninety years and over and 24 percent of those 85+, compared to 1 percent for persons aged sixty-five to seventy-four and 6 percent for those seventy-five to eighty-four years of age [4, 11]. The Agency for Health Care Policy and Research projects that just over half the women and one-third of the men who reached sixty-five in 1990 will be nursing home users. It is also estimated that by 2020, 1.7 million Americans aged sixty-five and over ultimately will be institutionalized [13].

The role of family and friends in fulfilling the long-term care needs of the frail elderly population has been well documented. There is no shortage of data pointing to the significance of informal support from spouses, children, other kin, friends, and neighbors in providing care to dependent older persons, care often credited with delaying or preventing costly institutionalization [14-17].

Factors other than the availability of support also affect the well-being of older persons. Among these are cultural values and expectations for caregiving, desire for independence and self-actualization on the part of the older person and the caregiver, and the costs associated with the caregiving role. Evidence is convincing that older persons place high value on their independence and that most elderly people in the United States prefer to remain in their own homes rather than share the home of a caregiver [18-21].

From the standpoint of the caregiver, evidence is equally persuasive that Americans tend to hold dear the happiness of the individual and their responsibility to spouse and children. Yet, the cultural ideal of taking care of one's parents, regardless of the sacrifice, remains clear and strong [21]. Combined with this conflict of values is a very real conflict of roles, particularly for middle-aged women [15, 16, 22, 23]. Moreover, many informal caregivers are themselves older than age sixty-five and report their health to be only fair or poor [18].

It is also evident that, for a small percentage of older persons (3-4%), no informal support systems exist [23, 24]. Many of these persons are childless and do not have that built-in emotional or instrumental support [25]. Current social trends portend an even greater number of childless elderly couples and individuals in the future. In addition, research shows that some people who have ongoing informal support still have considerable unmet needs [23, 26].

The need for long-term care is juxtaposed with the sky-rocketing costs of long-term care services. Nursing homes and other institutions that provide these services account for most of the national expenditures for long-term care. According to the Health Care Financing Administration, $59.9 billion was spent on nursing home care in 1991 [27], and that figure is projected to increase to $74.3 billion by 1993 [28].

Public support through Medicaid and Medicare provides over 50 percent of payments to nursing homes. In 1992, Medicaid paid 47.6 percent of the national cost for nursing home care [29]. However, 43 percent of that cost was paid for by residents and their families, and the cost of institutional care and the risk of impoverishment is high. The U.S. House of Representatives Select Committee on Aging [30] found that 90 percent of older people living alone who entered a nursing home depleted their savings within one year, and over 50 percent of elderly couples became impoverished within six months when one spouse became institutionalized.

## THE PUBLIC RESPONSE

Because of soaring costs, as well as the desire of most older persons who need long-term care to remain in their own homes, the demand has grown for care provided in the community rather than in institutions. Public programs that finance home and community-based long-term care services include Medicaid, Medicare, Older Americans Act initiatives, social services block grants, and initiatives run with general state revenues. While national expenditures for these programs remain limited compared to costs for institutional care, payments have quadrupled over the past decade. In 1992 public support from Medicaid and Medicare for community-based services totaled $9.4 billion [31].

One political response to the demand for increased long-term care services in the community was passage in 1981 of Section 2176 of the Omnibus Budget Reconciliation Act, which allowed states to request Medicaid waivers from the Health Care Financing Administration (HCFA) to provide a wide range of home and community-based services to Medicaid-eligible, impaired elderly persons [17]. These waivered programs are mandated to be targeted to persons who would otherwise meet the criteria for nursing home placement, and average per capita costs with the waiver are limited to average per capita costs without the waiver [32]. The primary objective of such programs is to delay or prevent institutionalization by providing in the home and community, coordinated programs of medical, social, and supportive services. While states vary in their commitment and capacities to provide home and community-based services, most states now offer at least limited coverage [33].

Central to program design is the concept of case management, where one individual or provider is responsible for assessment of client need and coordination of services [17]. Appropriate interaction between the services provided and existing informal networks of support is considered a crucial factor in the success of these community-based programs [34].

## THE CLIENT'S VOICE

Evaluation studies of a number of demonstration projects indicate that such programs are workable and accepted by elderly clients and their caregivers [34, 35]. For the most part, the existing research addressing their effectiveness is quantitative in design and generally has focused on objective outcomes, such as the cost-benefits of home care and various patient characteristics, including health status, mortality, institutionalization, met and unmet needs, as well as social and psychological well-being [33, 35-40]. Assessing the actual impact of these programs on chronically ill clients, however, presents certain difficulties. Studies examining mortality and various measures of health status generally have found little effect on recipients that could be attributed to program services [41]. Such findings are not unexpected since long-term care is concerned primarily with chronic illness, where improvement is often a distant prospect.

Research is scarce which reveals the perceptions of the care receivers themselves—the meanings they attach to the services provided and to their own abilities to cope with chronic illness, with and without help. Knowledge of the long-term care experiences of minority elders is particularly limited, despite the fact that minority status tends to increase the likelihood of chronic disease and disability. Jackson contends that the problems of aged minorities usually have been specified by individuals who are neither old nor members of minority groups [42]. She does not suggest that such aging specialists are not knowledgeable but that it is also important to have these elderly persons speak for themselves "if for no other reason than to understand more clearly the wide spectrum of problems [and] the reasons some aged persons who are objectively poor never consider themselves poverty stricken" [42, p. 202]. Certainly, some people who are deemed to be in poor health and functionally dependent, still consider themselves to be in relatively good health and independent [43, 44]. This sense of "relative privilege" dictates that the disabling effects of chronic conditions must be examined within the context of a complex relationship between social and health factors. As Keith states:

> Functionality itself has different meanings, and therefore must be measured differently in different cultural contexts. Depending on what is required for full social participation in various settings, and on the availability and cultural interpretation of social and physical supports, individuals with similar physical capabilities may be more or less able to function in different communities [43, p. 20].

Numerous researchers have contributed in-depth studies of various issues of old age, disability, and dependency and of particular settings where old people live. Matthews has explored the social world of old women, focusing on the management of identity in social relationships [45]. Kaufman examined the sources of meaning in old age and the construction of a sense of self throughout life [46]. Both of these authors dealt with the frequent need of old people to find ways to protect their self-image as mind and body deteriorate and dependency becomes a part of everyday life.

Other studies offer portrayals of age-segregated communities [47-49]. While the focus has been on the social organization and development of community within these settings, each work describes residents who, like the participants in our study, are struggling to maintain independence and remain in their communities. The research of Rubinstein and colleagues centers on frail elders who live alone and their perceptions of choice [20]. The message of this research is clear: holding on to autonomy and preserving control are key values. These authors underscore the importance for these old people of staying in their own homes where they have a modicum of control over their environment [20].

Several monographs provide in-depth views of frail elders who have had to leave their homes and enter nursing homes [50-54]. The most recent, *Old Friends,* is an account of Linda Manor and centers on the friendships that develop within the nursing home's walls [51]. Among these residents with multiple physical and mental ailments, Kidder finds evidence of the same continuing struggle for a meaningful identity in the midst of institutional dependency [51]. In *The Ends of Time,* Savishinsky analyzes the lives and experiences of residents, staff, and volunteers in what he calls a "good" nursing home [52]. The residents he describes also search for ways of handling their loss of autonomy and control. Some do whatever they can to retain a bit of power, even if it is only refusing to participate in planned activities.

In-depth portrayals of the non-institutional long-term care experiences of dependent older persons are in short supply. Two recent works attempt to fill this void in the home care literature-—*The Home Care Experience,* an edited volume by Gubrium and Sankar [55], and Gubrium's *The Mosaic of Care* [56]. These two volumes, however, concentrate on the caregiving arrangements, the impact on the caregiver, or the type of support network, rather than the perceptions and experiences of the dependent older person.

Few books on long-term care capture the feelings and emotions of the person receiving care. A notable exception is *Counting on Kindness* by Lustbader, a social worker, which speaks poignantly about the issues of power and dependency [57]. Lustbader weaves vignettes from the lives of her patients together with excerpts from literature to create a sensitive description of what it means to be dependent.

In *Kate Quinton's Days,* Sheehan offers a close-up view of one elderly woman's experience with the home care system in New York

City [58]. In her journalistic account, Sheehan describes Mrs. Quinton's hopes and frustrations about herself, about her daughters, and about the home care workers that float in and out of her life.

## AFRICAN AMERICAN VOICES

To date there has not been a clear look at the home care experience of older African Americans. Our research attempts to meet the need for recording and interpreting the ordinary life of elderly African Americans on their own terms, in their own surroundings, and, insofar as possible, in their own words. Our research is unique in two ways: it focuses on older people who are African American and poor, and it describes the viewpoint of care recipients and their relationships with the public programs designed to help them. This book provides an in-depth view of the experiences of these seven frail elders as both care receivers and as active participants in their own care. The two primary themes—the significant disabilities that often accompany old age and the tenacious will and ability to cope possessed by our informants—are reflected in the title: *Surviving Dependence*.

### Listening to Voices

Because a methodology was needed that could offer an in-depth view of the process of long-term care within its social context, ethnographic case study was selected [59]. Data were gathered during my year-long association with the seven older African Americans who allowed me to share their lives and witness their travails. All lived in a large metropolitan community and received long-term care services from Georgia's Community Care Services Program (CCSP), a Medicaid-waiver program established in 1982 by the Georgia General Assembly. The services provided by CCSP included: assessment and case management, home-delivered services (such as home health services and Meals-on-Wheels), alternative living services (where care is provided in a personal care home), adult day rehabilitation, respite care, emergency response, and homemaker services. The participants for the study were selected from clients served by a private, non-profit social service agency that, during the time of this research, contracted with CCSP to provide services. At that time, the agency served 299 clients, of whom 237 (78%) were aged sixty or over, 243 (83%) were female, and 197 (66%) were African American. According to program requirements, these individuals had sufficient disabling health problems to be certified for nursing home care.

The seven old people described in this book are kindred spirits in the common battles they wage, yet each situation has a uniqueness and each person a singular response to life. Consistent with naturalistic inquiry, individuals were selected not for their similarities but for the range of personal characteristics and experiences they reflect. They represent diverse living situations, a wide range of CCSP and informal services, and a variety of health problems and functional capacities. Six women and one man comprised the final sample. Four individuals lived alone, two with their families, and one woman shared her home with a roomer. Their level of physical disability extended from bedridden to ambulatory with aid of a walker; mental abilities ranged from moderate confusion to normal intellectual acuity.

The bulk of the data is drawn from regular observations and interviews with informants in their own homes. I watched their daily pastimes, and I talked to them about the people in their past and present lives and the meanings of activities and events. I observed caregivers as they provided their services and questioned them about their caregiving roles. While I watched and talked, I joined in typical at-home activities, such as watching TV, sitting, and performing occasional household and personal care tasks. Sometimes our associations led me down hospital corridors, through emergency rooms, and into grocery stores, pharmacies, doctors' offices, churches, emergency rooms, banks, and nursing homes. I observed how these frail elders negotiated other environments and interacted with auxiliary service providers.

## Researcher's Role

As our relationships developed, my involvement with each informant took on a unique character. In some cases my role leaned more toward that of an observer, while in others I became entwined in support networks. Sometimes I helped out as a way of reciprocating for their own willingness to share; other times I pitched in out of the necessity of the moment. Although each person offered me trust and affection, certain individuals were more needy and drew me closer. Because of my own "helping" nature, the difficulty for me was in preserving my objectivity and, where needs were especially great, resisting the urge to assume a major caregiver role. My sporadic contributions to their lives included meal preparation, laundry service, shopping, transportation, small gifts on holidays and birthdays, arranging for food stamps, filling out government forms, and, on one occasion, changing a diaper. Each person seemed grateful for my interest in them and their lives and, I hope, accepted me as their friend.

The personal and social attributes of the researcher are of central importance to those studied and affect the nature and kinds of data that can be collected [60]. While a number of well-respected naturalistic studies have been carried out by white researchers in black communities [61-66], a fair question nevertheless might be: how could a middle-aged, middle-class, white woman conduct a credible study of poor, African American elders? I have no doubt that my race was taken into account by informants and that being white restricted access to some information. However, my twenty years experience working in a low-income community center on behalf of older African Americans whose lives and problems parallel those of the study participants made me recognizably sympathetic, understanding, and unthreatening. In most cases we eventually found we shared friends and acquaintances. Although I could never fully experience the lives of these individuals, I came close enough to understand, and to present an accurate representation of, much of their feelings, motivations, and behaviors. In my mind, my racial identity was no more a problem than my age and social class.

In research, being a woman has advantages and disadvantages [60]. I believe my gender did restrict somewhat the personal information I was able to elicit from the one male informant. On the other hand, I think that being female and a homemaker was useful in relationships with female informants. Selecting a small number of informants whom I got to know very well permitted me to gain the necessary insight into their lives. While my viewpoint never will be identical to that of an old person or an African American (in this context, "insiders"), perhaps an "outsider's" view will add an additional and useful perspective [67].

Tammivaara and Enright's discussion of ways to elicit information from children is relevant, as a basic problem in research often is one of reducing status differences [68]. The fact that most observations and interviews took place on the informant's turf and that I was comfortable visiting in their homes seemed to make them feel at ease. Of greater significance, however, was their willingness to play the role of teacher to a receptive listener, in contrast to many of the people with whom they are in contact, who are less inclined to pay attention. As Tammivaara and Enright [68] espouse, I was able to convince these seven informants that not only was I sincerely interested in what they had to say, but I cared about them as individuals, a task I was able to accomplish because, following the advice of Lofland and Lofland [69], I "started where I was."

## Recording Voices

As is typical of naturalistic inquiry, the information was not collected to test specific hypotheses but to develop hypotheses pertaining to the cultural description portrayed. This analysis is an attempt to make sense of the data after the fact and to offer explanations about what was seen and heard. No generalizations will be made from these seven lives to the lives of other poor African American elders. Instead, whether a transfer to other situations can be made will be left to readers and future researchers to decide. Here we offer the *thick* description [70] that is crucial for making decisions about transferability.

The organization of the book is simple and straightforward. In Part I, we establish the social, cultural, and physical context of the long-term care experiences of these seven African American elders, beginning with the introduction of the informants. Since all seven are impaired physically, and some mentally, each is presented to the reader with a description of her/his health problems and disabling conditions. We allow the reader to look into their homes and neighborhoods, the settings for their long-term care experiences, and we describe relevant aspects of their life histories and their family ties.

We show how chronic conditions manifest themselves in a variety of troublesome symptoms that cause distress and limit these participants' social worlds and their abilities to perform basic tasks of daily living. We also begin to show how, despite these difficulties and guided by a strong value for independence, these impaired persons strive to take care of their own needs, using their remaining resources to develop strategies for self-care.

Part II describes the informal caregiving arrangements for each of these participants and provides understanding of how they view themselves as care receivers and how they relate to their informal caregivers. As the analysis proceeds, it becomes clear that the value placed upon preserving independence—to the fullest degree possible—has a major impact on the actions taken in these relationships, often creating barriers to effective care.

Building on this knowledge base, in Part III we turn to the complex formal system that delivers services to these clients, focusing on the role of services provided by the various types of aides. We discuss how these older African American clients evaluate the quality of the care they receive, and we examine their perceptions of the social and emotional aspects of the formal caregiving experience. Finally, we analyze the client's role in the formal caregiving process. We see that these clients are not just passive recipients of their formal services, but, rather, to the extent possible, are active participants in the process of care.

The concluding section of the book (Part IV) is devoted to a discussion of the implications of our findings for future research and for the development of long-term care policy and programs. We offer strategies for providing care that enable providers to gain greater understanding of the care receiver's situation, to take into account the care receiver's point of view, and to build their programs around the roles that care receivers prefer.

In the Epilogue we revisit the seven participants to bring the reader up to date about what has transpired in their lives since the completion of the research.

## REFERENCES

1. K. Markides, *Aging and Heath: Perspectives on Race, Ethnicity and Class,* Sage Publications, Inc., Newbury Park, California, 1989.
2. C. F. Longino, Jr., G. Warheit, and J. A. Green, Class, Aging and Health, in *Aging and Health: Perspectives on Race, Ethnicity and Class,* K. Markides (ed.), Sage Publications, Inc., Newbury Park, California, pp. 79-110, 1989.
3. K. G. Manton, L. S. Corder, and E. Stallard, Estimates of Change in Chronic Disability and Institutional Incidence and Prevalence Rates in the U. S. Elderly Population from the 1982, 1984, and 1989 National Long Term Care Survey, *Journal of Gerontology: Social Sciences, 48*:4, pp. S153-S166, 1993.
4. American Association of Retired Persons and U.S. Administration on Aging, *A Profile of Older Americans:1993,* Washington, D. C., 1993.
5. P. L. Dressel, Gender, Race and Class in Later Life, *The Gerontologist, 28*:2, pp. 177-180, 1988.
6. J. J. Jackson and C. Perry, Physical Health Conditions of Middle-Aged and Aged Blacks, in *Aging and Health: Perspectives on Race, Ethnicity and Class*, K. Markides (ed.), Sage Publications, Inc., Newbury Park, California, pp. 111-176, 1989.
7. J. J. Jackson, Race, National Origin, Ethnicity and Aging, in *Handbook of Aging and the Social Sciences*, R. H. Binstock and E. Shanas (eds.) (2nd Edition), Van Nostrand Reinhold, New York, pp. 264-303, 1985.
8. R. C. Manuel and M. L. Berk, A Look at Similarities and Differences in Older Minority Populations, *Aging,* pp. 21-29, 1983.
9. J. Van Nostrand, *Health Data on Older Americans*, United States Public Health Service, Series 3, No. 27, 1993.
10. B. W. K. Yee and G. D. Weaver, Ethnic Minorities and Health Promotion: Developing a "Culturally Competent Agenda," *Generations, XVIII*:1, pp. 39-44, 1994.
11. C. M. Murtaugh, P. Kemper, and B. C. Spillman, The Risk of Nursing Home Use in Later Life, *Medical Care, 28*:10, pp. 952-962, 1990.

12. American Association of Retired Persons, *Building a Better Health Care System: America's Challenge of the 1990s*, Washington, D. C., 1990.

13. Agency for Health Care Policy and Research, *Nonreimbursed Home Health Care: Beyond the Bills*, Washington, D. C., 1990.

14. E. Shanas, Social Myth As Hypothesis: The Case of Family Relations of Old People, *The Gerontologist, 19*, pp. 3-9, 1979.

15. M. Cantor, Strain Among Caregivers: A Study of Experience in the United States, *The Gerontologist, 23*, pp. 597-604, 1983.

16. R. Montgomery and K. Kosloski, A Longitudinal Analysis of Nursing Home Placement for Dependent Elders Cared for by Spouses versus Adult Children, *Journal of Gerontology: Social Sciences, 49*, pp. S62-S74, 1994.

17. J. McCann, Long-term Home Care for the Elderly: Perceptions of Nurses, Physicians, and Primary Caregivers, *QRB,18*, pp. 66-74, 1988.

18. E. Shanas, Older People and their Families: The New Pioneers, *Journal of Marriage and the Family, 42*, pp. 9-15, 1980.

19. C. Fry, *Aging in Culture and Society: Comparative Viewpoints and Strategies*, J. R. Bergin, Brooklyn, 1980.

20. R. L. Rubinstein, J. C. Kilbride, and S. Nagy, *Elders Living Alone*, Aldine de Gruyter, New York, 1992.

21. R. Kalish, Of Children and Grandfathers: A Speculative Essay on Dependence, *The Gerontologist, 7*, pp. 65-79, 1967.

22. E. Brody, "Women in the Middle" and Family Help to Older People, *The Gerontologist, 21*, pp. 471-480, 1981.

23. J. Morris and S. Sherwood, Informal Support Resources for Vulnerable Elderly Persons: Can They Be Counted On, Why Do They Work? *International Journal of Aging and Human Development, 18*, pp. 81-98, 1984.

24. E. Stoller and L. Earl, Help with Activities of Everyday Life: Sources of Support for the Non-institutionalized Elderly, *The Gerontologist, 23*, pp. 64-69, 1983.

25. N. G. Choi, Patterns and Determinants of Social Service Utilization: Comparison of the Childless Elderly and Elderly Parents Living with or Apart from their Children, *The Gerontologist, 34*:3, pp. 353-362, 1994.

26. E. P. Stoller and K. L. Pugliesi, Size and Effectiveness of Informal Helping Networks: A Panel Study of Older People in the Community, *Journal of Health and Social Behavior, 32*:3, pp. 180-191, 1991.

27. S. W. Letsch, H. C. Lazenby, K. R. Levit, and C. A. Cowan, National Health Expenditures, 1991, *Health Care Financing Review, 14*:2, pp. 1-30, 1992.

28. Health Care Financing Administration, Bureau of Data Management and Strategy, *1993 HCFA Statistics*, HCFA Pub. No. 03341, June 1993.

29. American Health Care Association, *A Proposal for Long Term Care Financing Reform*, Washington, D. C., 1993.

30. U.S. House of Representatives Select Committee on Aging, Long-Term Care and Personal Impoverishment: Seven in Eleven Elderly Living Alone Are at Risk, U.S. Congress, October 1987.

31. U.S. General Accounting Office, *Long-Term Care: Status of Quality Assurance and Measurement in Home and Community-Based Services*,

Report to the Chairman, Committee on Finance, U.S. Senate, Washington, D. C., March 1994.

32. P. Doty, K. Liu, and J. Wiener, An Overview of Long-Term Care, *Health Care Financing Review, 6*, pp. 69-78, 1985.

33. Administration on Aging, Infrastructure of Home and Community Based Services for Functionally Impaired Elderly, *State Source Book*, U.S. Department of Health and Human Services, 1994.

34. K. B. Haskins, J. Capitman, F. Colligen, B. Degraaf, and C. Yordi, *Evaluation of Community Long-Term Care Demonstration Projects: Extramural Report*, Health Care Financing Administration, Baltimore, 1987.

35. P. Kemper, R. Brown, G. Carcagno, R. Applebaum, J. Christianson, W. Carson, S. Dunstan, T. Granneman, M. Harrigan, N. Holden, R. Phillips, J. Schore, C. Thornton, J. D. Wooldridge, and F. Skidmore, *The Evaluation of the National Long-term Care Demonstrations Final Report*, Mathematica Policy Research, Inc., Princeton, New Jersey, 1986.

36. S. Sherwood and J. Morris, The Pennsylvania Domiciliary Care Experiment: 1. Impact on Quality of Life, *American Journal of Public Health, 73*, pp. 646-653, 1983.

37. W. Weissert, C. Cready, and J. Pawelak, The Past and Future of Community-based Long-term Care, *The Milbank Quarterly, 66*, pp. 309-388, 1988.

38. K. Braun and C. Rose, The Hawaii Geriatric Foster Care Experiment: Impact Evaluation and Cost Analysis, *The Gerontologist, 26*, pp. 515-524, 1986.

39. D. Challis and C. Davies, Home Care of the Frail Elderly in the United Kingdom: Matching Resources to Needs, *Home Health Care Services Quarterly, 5*, pp. 89-109, 1985.

40. T. Wan, W. Weissert, and R. Livieratos, Geriatric Daycare and Homemaker Services: An Experimental Study, *Journal of Gerontology, 35*, pp. 256-274, 1980.

41. M. Linn and B. Linn, Qualities of Institutional Care that Affect Outcome, *Aged Care and Services Review, 2*, pp. 1-13, 1980.

42. J. J. Jackson, *Minorities and Aging*, Wadsworth Publishing Co., Belmont, California, 1980.

43. J. Keith, *Old People As People: Social and Cultural Influences on Aging and Old Age*, Little, Brown, Boston, 1982.

44. T. Wan and W. Weissert, Social Support Networks, Patient Status and Institutionalization, *Research on Aging, 3*, pp. 240-256, 1981.

45. S. Matthews, *The Social World of Old Women: Management of Self-Identity*, Sage Publications Inc., Beverly Hills, California, 1979.

46. S. Kaufman, *The Ageless Self: Sources of Meaning in Late Life*, The University of Wisconsin Press, Madison, Wisconsin, 1986.

47. A. Hochschild, *The Unexpected Community*, Prentice Hall, Englewood Cliffs, New Jersey, 1973.

48. J. K. Ross, *Old People, New Lives: Community Creation in a Retirement Residence*, University of Chicago Press, Chicago, 1977.

49. J. Smithers, *Determined Survivors: Community Life Among the Urban Elderly*, Rutgers University Press, New Brunswick, New Jersey, 1985.
50. J. Gubrium, *Living and Dying at Murray Manor*, St. Martin's, New York, 1975.
51. T. Kidder, *Old Friends*, Houghton-Mifflin Co., New York, 1993.
52. J. Savishinsky, *The Ends of Time: Life and Work in a Nursing Home*, Bergin and Garvey, New York, 1991.
53. R. Shield, *Uneasy Endings: Daily Life in an American Nursing Home*, Cornell University Press, Ithaca, New York, 1988.
54. M. O'Brien, *Anatomy of a Nursing Home: A New View of Residential Life*, National Health Publishing, Owings Mills, Maryland, 1989.
55. J. F. Gubrium and A. Sankar (eds.), *The Home Care Experience*, Sage Publications, Inc., Newbury Park, California, 1990.
56. J. F. Gubrium, *The Mosaic of Care*, Springer, New York, 1991.
57. W. Lustbader, *Counting on Kindness: The Dilemmas of Dependency*, The Free Press, New York, 1991.
58. S. Sheehan, *Kate Quinton's Days*, New American Library, New York, 1984.
59. S. B. Merrimam, *Case Study Research in Education: A Qualitative Approach*, Jossey-Bass Publishers, San Francisco, 1988.
60. R. M. Emerson, *Contemporary Field Research: A Collection of Readings*, Waveland Press, Prospect Heights, Illinois, 1983.
61. E. Liebow, *Tally's Corner: A Study of Negro Streetcorner Men*, Little, Brown, Boston, 1967.
62. W. H. Whyte, *Street Corner Society*, University of Chicago Press, Chicago, 1955.
63. C. Stack, *All Our Kin*, Harper and Row, New York, 1974.
64. U. Hannerz, *Soulside: Inquiries into Ghetto Culture and Community*, Columbia University Press, New York, 1969.
65. M. C. Dougherty, *Becoming a Woman in Rural Black Culture*, Holt, Rinehart and Winston, New York, 1978.
66. J. Aschenbrenner, *Lifelines: Black Families in Chicago*, Holt, Rinehart, and Winston, New York, 1975.
67. R. K. Merton, Insiders and Outsiders: A Chapter in the Sociology of Knowledge, in *A History of Sociological Analysis*, T. Bottomore and R. Nisbet (eds.), Basic Books, New York, pp. 9-46, 1978.
68. J. Tammivaara and D. S. Enright, On Eliciting Information: Dialogues with Child Informants, *Anthropology and Education Quarterly, 17*, pp. 218-238, 1986.
69. J. Lofland and L. H. Lofland, *Analyzing Social Settings: A Guide to Qualitative Observation and Analysis* (2nd Edition), Wadsworth Publishing Co., Belmont, California, 1984.
70. C. Geertz, Thick Description: Toward an Interpretative Theory of Culture, in *Contemporary Field Research*, R. M. Emerson (ed.), Waveland Press, Prospect Heights, Illinois, 1983.

# Part I
# The Context of Care

# CHAPTER
1

# Meeting the Participants

At the beginning of each day, Mr. Avant removes the padlock from the inside of Eloise Little's bedroom door. The main entrance to their home is through the living room, but Mrs. Little's visitors enter from the front screened-in porch through this door directly into her bedroom, which is her world. Upon entering, the signs of illness and impairment are immediately apparent. The room is usually darkened, the curtains drawn, the only light emitting from the small black and white TV. It is very warm, summer or winter, and the smells of urine or feces are often unmistakable. These days Mrs. Little is always in bed, a double bed with a big wooden head-board. She either sits or lies slumped over on one side, sometimes sipping on a bottle of beer from a straw. She has trouble finding a comfortable position, unable to straighten out her misshapen body, and she appears even smaller than her ninety pounds, her frail bones covered with just skin. She drapes her shoulders with a small blanket or towel, the button which controls her emergency response system is around her neck, and sometimes her balding head is hooded with a cap she has made out of an old pajama leg. Her body rests on several layers of brown paper bags or commercial bed pads, to protect her bed from urine. Some days Mrs. Little is groggy from the beer, drifting in and out of sleep, but on other days her eyes are bright and lively, and she is eager to talk, about her neglectful family or about better days when she could take care of herself.

Mrs. Little is one of the seven African American elders you will come to know in this book. While she is the oldest and most impaired of these participants, the reality of old age and chronic disability is at the core of each life. It is a reality beset by nagging symptoms, gradual decline, and permanence. Aging for them has become a one-way journey toward total dependence.

17

These seven elders have much in common. Like many old people, they have multiple chronic conditions, including arthritis, hypertension, heart disease, diabetes, urinary dysfunction, organic and affective brain disorders, alcoholism, and hearing and visual impairments. These conditions are manifested in different ways and to different degrees, yet they result in the dependence of each of them on others to meet many or most of their basic needs.

They are all poor and have lived in poverty most or all of their lives. Their annual incomes, now derived from a combination of Social Security benefits and Supplemental Security Income (SSI), are below $5000. Only one person maintains a savings account that approaches the SSI resource limit of $2000. The other six have little or no cash savings.

Like many African Americans of their generation who have lived in the South, they have a history of struggle. Because of racism and poverty they have had limited opportunities for education, employment, housing, and health care. Being black and poor has increased their chances of experiencing chronic disease and disability. We see throughout this book how race and poverty affect their lives and their abilities to care for themselves and to get the additional care they need.

All seven live in high crime areas where much of the housing is substandard, and residences are interspersed with businesses, vacant lots, and boarded-up houses. As is typical of most poor areas, the businesses that remain are characterized by high prices and low quality and include no pharmacies or supermarkets. The lack of convenient services as well as the prevalence of crime further reduce the possibilities for retaining independence.

Despite many similarities, the homes of these seven participants remain distinct. Four people live in privately-owned, single-family dwellings, one in a large public housing complex, and two in public highrises for the elderly. While all homes have been adapted in some ways to accommodate disability—special equipment purchased, ramps built, rooms rearranged—in each setting barriers remain that impede both the ability of the older person to function independently and the ability of others to provide care. For those who own their own houses, maintenance, even a minor repair, is often an insurmountable financial undertaking. No resources are available for cosmetic renovation, and rarely can they make structural changes to improve the accessibility of their houses, and thus their suitability as residences for impaired older people.

The importance of the place where one lives takes on increased significance when one has little opportunity to escape its confines. As the disabilities of these individuals have increased over the years, their lifespaces have diminished accordingly. Except on rare occasions they are bound to their homes. Mrs. Little's frontier, for example, extends no further than the end of her bed. In some homes the accoutrements of illness can be relegated to the "backstage" [1] of day-to-day life, but in other situations the evidence of disease and disability is unmistakable. These life spaces reflect the physical and mental states of the occupants, their resources for support, and their positions in society. As Rubinstein found in his study of frail elders, when space diminishes with increasing age and infirmity, the home or personal environment may become an expression of self [2]. So we see Mrs. Little's identity reflected in her personal environment, the world around her bed, with all the artifacts of her now-constricted life. We recognize the objects and events that give meaning to her life, as we identify her despair and neglect. Each of these seven homes reveals equally telling clues about the identity of each frail tenant.

Matthews, in her study of the social world of old women, discussed the subjective meanings attached to the settings in which people lead their lives [3]. She noted that people's self-identities are affected by their feelings about their settings and emphasized the importance for older women of feeling "at home" in the world around them in terms of familiarity with physical aspects of settings and the people who share them. Familiar settings are considered valuable assets because familiarity contributes to a subjective sense of belonging and allows the world around to be taken for granted, providing order. The homes of the old people in this book may not always be safe, comfortable, or convenient, but for each person, remaining in these familiar settings is a primary value. Staying at home enables them to retain some of the control that seems to slip away so quickly with dependence.

With declining abilities, however, the challenges of home environments can become overwhelming. Familiarity does not compensate for doors that do not accommodate wheelchairs or bathtubs that defy arthritic limbs. Lawton and Nahemow have proposed that individuals adapt better to the exigencies of aging when they maintain a congruence between two factors—environmental press and competence—that is, when the demands of their home environments closely match their own abilities [4]. Some of these participants no longer are able to sustain this steady state.

The introduction to these seven African American elders focuses on their disabling conditions, their life histories, and the physical settings in which they now live their constricted lives. Although each person embodies a lifetime of unique experiences and relationships, through each life the common threads of disease and disability and of race and poverty are interwoven. In each life these traits are a commanding force.

## ELOISE LITTLE

Mrs. Little is eighty-seven years old. She is an alcoholic and suffers from malnutrition, hypertension, congestive heart failure, severe osteoarthritis, some urinary dysfunction, and gout. Her condition has steadily deteriorated over the last several years, her weight dropping from 150 to 90 pounds. Her symptoms are many and severe. She is no longer able to get out of bed, turn over on her own, or stand, even with assistance. Because she has no one to provide regular care, she must use an indwelling catheter and wear diapers. During the past year, Mrs. Little has been hospitalized three times, once for dehydration and malnutrition and twice for urinary tract infections, probably the result of her catheter. Although her alcohol consumption causes confusion and grogginess, she is generally lucid, and the reality of her hopeless condition often creates intense anxiety:

> I'm half dead now. I've been sick for years, not down like I am now, just draggin'. Oh yeah, I had big arms, legs. My legs gone, my stomach gone, jaws done sunk in, look like I have false teeth. I'm bad sick. I'm so weak. I ain't got the strength of a buzzard. I know one thing: I can't turn over to save my life. I've been in misery a long time. I got the arthritis all over. I be hurtin' from my toes to my head. It be all over me like somebody nailin' on me. It hurts like someone hit you on it when you turn over. I'm stiff. My knees is stiff. I'm weak in my knees and back. The older I get, the weaker I get. I done worried so much 'til I ain't got good sense no more. I'm crazy as a betsy bug.

As Mrs. Little states, being sick is not a new experience. Six years ago she fell off a foot stool in her highrise and injured her knee. She remembers "waking up in a nursing home," where she remained for six months, an experience still vivid in her memory:

> Cruelest people you ever saw. Treated you worse than a mad dog. Laid messed up all day and night. Passed by you like you weren't even there.

Mrs. Little finally was able to persuade her sister, Rozena, to take her out of the nursing home and into her own home, but a year later Rozena died, leaving Mrs. Little again alone.

Born and raised in the city, Mrs. Little admits to a sometimes colorful past, rarely passing up a good fight and even getting "locked-up" on occasion. She was "the baby" in a family of three girls and one boy and is now the only one still living. She had two husbands, but they are deceased. She lived with the second one for twenty-five years, until his death in 1960, after a long illness. She said they "got along like cats and dogs at first, but then it turned around." She was alone with him when he died: "He grabbed both my hands, smiled, and shook his head. They had to prise his hands off of me."

When she was "real young," before she married, Mrs. Little had one child, a son. Her sisters helped raise him, but while he was still a young man he moved to New York, and over the years Mrs. Little lost track of him and assumes he is now dead. Her only living relatives are a half-brother and sister in the city and three "in the country" (about 50 miles away), two nieces and a nephew.

Born into poverty, Mrs. Little began earning a living as a teenager, "ironing in white folks' houses and taking care of little ones, them that could walk." She talks with pride of ironing clothes so stiff one could "hear them coming" and of "saving many a child from a whipping."

The house where Mrs. Little now lives has been her home only for the last six years, beginning when her sister brought her there from the nursing home. It has been in her family, however, for over seventy-five years, and at one time, the neighbors say, it was kept in top shape, but since the sister's death five years ago it has been left to deteriorate. Mrs. Little now shares her home with Mr. Avant, a roomer, who moved in three years ago after losing his job at age sixty-two.

Because she is bedridden and often alone, the arrangement of Mrs. Little's world is crucial. Her door is left unlocked during daylight hours to allow entry to any helpers, and she keeps all the items she needs each day within her reach, most of them on the bed. Her heating pad, always on, is right beside her, as is her special "wire," a bent coat hanger she uses to reach or arrange things. Several plastic baskets contain such essentials as a letter opener, a salt shaker, fingernail scissors, a pen, a beer opener, small gifts visitors have brought, bottles of medicine, her special brand of medicated soap, plastic drinking straws, and phone numbers of family and friends. Mrs. Little worries about her possessions disappearing, keeping as many as possible within her range of vision, and she insists that the baskets be arranged "her" way, sitting on a particular green towel. Under the covers, under the green towel, she keeps her foodstamps and a small change purse. The bulk of her money she pins inside her nightgown for safekeeping. Other signs of her day-to-day life are found on top of her bed—one or two aluminum foil containers of food, assorted packages of bread, or cartons of milk from the home-delivered meal program, and a large blue stack of protective pads for her bed.

Other necessities are close to the bed and still within reach. On one side sit the portable commode, the waste basket, a small table for the phone, and her spit can (for snuff). On the other side, another table holds a pitcher of water, a glass, a can of snuff, a large plastic pig for pennies, and the control box for her emergency response system. Mrs. Little keeps right beside her on the floor her beer, in a brown paper bag, her pocketbook with all of her important papers, and several plastic bags of assorted clothing.

Also in the cramped bedroom, but out of Mrs. Little's reach, are two dressers—the tops spread with an array of liniments and lotions—a chifforobe, the television, an electric three-wheeled cart, two chairs for visitors, and, in the corner, a large metal wash tub to catch the rain water that leaks through the roof. A tiny refrigerator, just large enough to hold a few leftover meals and cartons of juice, sits next to a toaster oven, on top of an old metal cabinet used to store canned food and other staples. On the mantle are Mrs. Little's family pictures. Her "street" clothes hang on the back of the door. The room is typically dirty and in disarray. Mice often scamper around, and at night rats have been known to venture even onto her bed.

The heater that warms Mrs. Little's bedroom is located in the living room, an arrangement that contributes to high heating bills in colder months. In this room and in the dining room the furniture is piled to one side to avoid water leaks and collapsing ceilings. Only the rooms Mr. Avant uses—his bedroom, the kitchen and the bathroom—are clean and tidy.

In some ways the arrangement of Mrs. Little's environment increases the burdens of providing her care. When Mr. Avant leaves the house, he always padlocks the door to the large refrigerator where his food is stored, to prevent access by Mrs. Little's alcoholic nephew. Sometimes he even locks the door to the kitchen, thus barring would-be caregivers from this room and the bathroom, the only sources of water to bathe Mrs. Little. Neither the washing machine nor the oven is in working order.

Mrs. Little's house sits atop a steep hill with two sets of steps leading down to the street. While a concrete ramp leads from the back door to the driveway, the driveway has deteriorated to the point where it is now impassable for a wheelchair or even a car. The houses on either side are occupied, and an elementary school and church are across the street, increasing somewhat the safety of her immediate area. A small grocery store and a laundromat, each with irregular hours, are located within the block.

## RUBY WASHINGTON

> I'm a diabetes person. My blood is high. It's been like that ever since my legs got off. I can't see very well, can't see out of my right eye. I take my glasses off and lay 'em down and can't find 'em. I get where I can't hear so good. I'm just weak in my back. When my leg is swollen, I can't walk. Since I had my second leg off, I got in the chair, but when I had one leg off, I didn't have the chair. I put my leg on and I had a walking stick and I could go anywhere I wanted—go to the store, out in the yard. I could go anywhere. I got up walking yesterday with Jones and my nurse. The doctor said for me not to walk too much, said I press against my heart and that wasn't good for me. The doctor said it wouldn't hurt for me to walk in the house and do things, but it wouldn't do for me to try to get out and walk in the streets. I wished I *could* walk around the house by myself, but he said he want somebody to be with me at all times.

At age eighty-five, Ruby Washington's physical disabilities are compelling. Both legs have been amputated at the knee, the result of her diabetic condition, and she has hypertension, angina, urinary dysfunction, and some visual and hearing loss. Although able, with difficulty, to transfer from her bed to her wheelchair, to propel her own chair with her hands, and to walk with assistance around the house wearing her protheses, she, like Mrs. Little, spends most of her time in bed.

Mrs. Washington is one of six children, the oldest of four remaining siblings. She alone of the seven participants never worked outside the home, but was supported by her husband until his death twenty years ago. She still lives in the home where she and her husband raised their four children, but she now shares it with her son, Robert, and Mr. Jones, her common-law husband. Another son and a daughter live in Philadelphia; her other daughter was shot and killed several years ago in a domestic dispute.

Mrs. Washington's home is surrounded on three sides by vacant lots and abandoned houses; a popular liquor store abuts her backyard; and the nearby street corner, as well as the adjacent vacant lot, are neighborhood hangouts. Robert, her son, runs an informal liquor house from his quarters, and, when he is at home, patrons frequently gather on the front porch, drinking from paper cups. At night Mrs. Washington sometimes hears rocks hit the side of her house, and she is afraid to stay at home alone. Recently, she was awakened by a night-time intruder who left with her pocketbook and her Social Security check.

Like Mrs. Little, Mrs. Washington also keeps her door unlocked during daylight hours, and visitors enter directly from the front porch into the living room, which also serves as her bedroom. Soft spoken and always pleasant, Mrs. Washington sits surrounded by those items indispensable to her daily routine—the telephone, radio, bedpan, pocketbook, thick glasses, and comb. Again the scent of urine assaults the senses. She is dressed, at least from the waist up; a towel in her lap covers the stumps of her legs. Mr. Jones customarily sits on the sofa watching TV or out on the front porch. Clues to Mrs. Washington's disabled state are conspicuous—the regulation hospital bed with the trapeze-like pull-bar suspended overhead, Mrs. Washington's protheses standing in the corner, and her medications and bedpan nearby.

Here, too, the setting is dreary, signaling inattention as well as poverty. The room where Mrs. Washington spends her time is shabby and unkept with thick dust and cobwebs in the corners and roaches scaling the soiled and faded drapes. With no dressers or closets for storage, clothes are stored by the side of the bed in large plastic trash bags and hanging on the backs of the doors. The sofa shows the long years of wear, a large non-functioning television serves as a table, and the only source of heat, a gas space heater, is installed in the old fireplace. The room is brightened only by a single lightbulb suspended over Mrs. Washington's bed, a few scattered decorations, and a faded portrait of Martin Luther King, Jr. hanging from the crumbling plaster walls. Thick wire screen is nailed over the windows for defense.

Mrs. Washington's house has steadily deteriorated since her husband's death. Like Mrs. Little, she has had problems with a leaky roof and recently contracted to have "a new top" put on her house for $1500, paying $127 per month out of her small check of $427. The stove and refrigerator are antiquated and barely functioning, and she has no washing machine, only an old-fashioned kitchen sink.

Because her house is all on one level, Mrs. Washington is able to wheel herself from the front room back to the kitchen, but not into the bathroom, where the door is too narrow, or out to the street. Although a makeshift ramp leads down from the back porch, no pathway extends around to the sidewalk in front, making it impossible for her to leave home without assistance.

## VIOLA WORTH

Viola Worth, aged seventy-five, is the least impaired of this group of African American elders. She has mobility problems, resulting from life-long scoliosis (abnormal curvature of the spine), arthritis, and the recent replacement of a diseased hip, and, although able to walk with the aid of a walker, she tires easily and frequently uses her wheelchair to get around her house. In addition, she has minor cardiovascular, digestive, and urinary problems. Over the years she has learned to accommodate her limitations:

> Listen, in my mind, my main trouble is the condition I been had all my life [scoliosis]. My body is twisted all kind of ways. You know, down through the years it's gonna affect you. That's one thing. I know I'm gonna have arthritis. So in my mind my main condition is my arthritis and my handicap I been had all my life. My main thing in my book is I don't let the arthritis worry me. I think the handicap I was born with is the main thing that affect me.

Ms. Worth grew up in the country on a sharecropping farm. Her mother died when she was six years old, an indelible event in her life:

> My mother called me to her bedside when she died. She turned over and said, "Mama's going away. I want you to be a good girl. You going to have a hard time when I'm gone." I'll never forget that. I asked the Lord to give me strength.

After her mother's death, Ms. Worth was raised by an aunt, but she remembers more affirmatively the white children on the farm who were her friends and her white "goddaddy" who protected her from her aunt's frequent abuse:

> Most of my friends were white. My goddaddy was white. My god-daddy told her [her aunt] if she didn't treat his little crippled girl right, he would put the Ku Klux Klan on her. That's the first I ever heard of the Klan. He'd get her if she got too rough on me. He taken up for me.

When she was thirteen, Ms. Worth went to live with a white family to take care of the children, while "still a child herself." A few years later she had her own child, a son, but in 1937 she left him with relatives and moved to the city with the family for whom she was working. Ms. Worth was then twenty-one years old, and she continued to make her living taking care of children until well into her sixties. Now she supplements her fixed income selling cold drinks to friends and neighbors, as well as parking spaces on the adjacent vacant lot for events at a nearby stadium.

Except for sporadic periods when she lived "on the lot" (in the back of the homes of white families she worked for), Ms. Worth has resided at her present address since 1945, the year she moved in to take care of an ailing "Auntie." Save for occasional borders, she has lived alone since her aunt's death in 1965. Although she is presently estranged from her son and granddaughter and has contact with no other blood relatives, Ms. Worth has many friends and adopted kin that, for her, take the place of true kin. She never married.

Ms. Worth's home is located in the same high-crime neighborhood as Mrs. Washington's, and it, too, is surrounded by vacant houses and lots. On the outside her house blends in with the run-down appearance of the area, but on the inside, it is comfortable, neat, clean, and attractively furnished, albeit with many worn, taped-together, or secondhand items. The visiting areas reveal few signs of her impaired state, and, in contrast to the homes of the two women described previously, her home is pleasant, with a cared-for look about it. The house has six rooms—three bedrooms (one very tiny), a living room, dining room, and kitchen—and one bath, with a porch, one half of which is screened, across the front.

Ms. Worth spends most of her time in her bedroom, the living room, or the kitchen, keeping the other rooms closed off, except in the summer when she sometimes takes refuge in the small room in the back where it is cooler. She greets visitors warmly at the door, using her walker rather than the wheelchair, unless she is "extra stiff," and is always neatly dressed, customarily in pants and a T-shirt, her short gray hair in gheri-curls. Visitors sit in the "front room," the living room, where there is a sofa, three comfortable chairs, a large color TV, a corner cabinet filled with sparkling crystal and china, and several tables, which prominently display pictures and mementos of her numerous "play children" and friends. Only in the bedroom, where fresh, brightly colored linens adorn the bed, are there signs of Ms. Worth's impaired condition—a portable commode next to her bed, a paraffin bath (to soak arthritic hands and feet) against the wall, and various medicines, liniments, and lotions lined up on the dresser.

The physical layout of Ms. Worth's house allows her to be mobile, even in her present partially ambulatory condition. All doorways are sufficiently wide for her wheelchair, and space is adequate for maneuvering throughout. Numerous steep steps bar her access to the street from her front door, but the back door is at ground level, and a paved walk reaches almost up to the driveway. She keeps the yard surrounding her house maintained, and, even though the ground is obstructed with rocks and tree roots, Ms. Worth is able to slowly make her way on her walker from the front to the back and even down to the street.

Although Ms. Worth depends on her regular benefits to cover her basic needs, her informal businesses allow her to make non-essential purchases from time to time:

> That little change helps out. Well, I don't just spend it because I have it. Just kind of hold to it 'cause I have other things I can use it for. That's the reason I maybe have a little change most of the time. Like when parking come, I be able to have a little change on hand. I don't just depend on it. The only thing I have to depend on is my monthly salary [her government benefits]. I know I didn't have none saved up, like leaning on or pinching on. I just be thankful 'cause whatever I get, I budget myself.

Unlike the other participants, because of this "extra change," Ms. Worth is able to treat herself to a new set of sheets or a used lamp from the thrift store and over the years has purchased several new appliances on the installment plan, such as a washing machine, refrigerator, freezer, stove, and two color televisions.

These extras do not, however, stretch to major home repairs, but Ms. Worth budgets her meager resources as best she can to keep her house at least "patched up":

> I ain't able to have my house pulled up or have things done like I want to, but the main little things. Just like my screen out there, I done that the time I wasn't paying gas. I still owe him a little bit on it. I called the man to look at it 'cause I wanted it either fixed or all that stuff tore out. The house look bad enough. It makes your house look bad and make me feel bad. I like to get somebody to really get some work done 'cause I ain't able to do it. Ain't no need in soaking the house to do it. Got to get patched up and patched up. They might could break it down so I could pay it with my little money, but it would take so long I might be dead and in heaven or torment or somewhere, and then the house would be all in debt, and then the next thing you know they been torn it down and I'd still be in debt. So, I just keep it patched up.

## REVEREND JOSEPH SCOTT

Also wheelchair-bound, Rev. Scott, the youngest participant at age seventy-one, suffers from severe rheumatoid arthritis and skeletal trauma, resulting from a car accident when in his forties. Poor circulation, caused by his arthritic condition, makes the healing of wounds difficult, and during the past year he has been hospitalized twice for skin grafts on his legs, attempts to heal chronic skin ulcers. Because of these ulcers, Rev. Scott has been unable to walk or drive his car for over a year, and his arthritic hands limit his ability to perform manual tasks. He can, however, maneuver around his house with ease and onto his back porch in his battery-powered wheelchair. Despite his significant physical impairments, Rev. Scott has weathered his disabling condition now for many years, and, like Ms. Worth, he has adjusted to his limitations and still has hopes of getting better:

> Well, as far as my health is concerned, I don't feel sick. My biggest problem is this leg, going to the clinic and staying awhile in the hospital. I haven't been able to get up and walk lately. I'd like to do that. Last time I tried to walk, it started bleeding. I'm anxious for it to heal up so I can start back exercising. Not too much pain, just one little spot kind of have an edge on it. I feel the effects of the arthritis. Staying in the hospital and keeping the "unaboot" on [a cast-like bandage that is changed only every couple of weeks], and not taking my exercises like I should, I'm beginning to feel that arthritis becoming active. I've had a flare up every so often, every two or three years. Some of them are worse than others.

While none of the women portrayed in this book went beyond the elementary grades, Rev. Scott finished three years of college, an accomplishment that is a testament to his many strengths. One of eleven children in a sharecropper's family, the oldest of the three boys, he has early memories of working on the farm. Because his help was needed at home, until the last two years in high school, he only attended school from October through March, and when he was seventeen, his father died, leaving him with the responsibility of managing the farm and supporting the family. Rev. Scott remembers learning how to pray during those difficult times:

> Times were not always good then. I would hunt to put food on the table. I had a big load on my shoulders. I kind of learned how to pray. I asked the Lord to make it possible for my brothers and sisters to have a fair chance in life.

When his youngest brother (now an artist and college professor) was five years old, Rev. Scott went off to the city to college, continuing to work and send money home to his mother. He met his future wife while singing in the church choir and dropped out of school to marry her, later becoming a successful building contractor and Baptist minister.

But fate intervened when Rev. Scott was struck by a car in front of his house at the age of forty, and his frequent hospitalizations over the next few years depleted his savings and left him with only his house and car, help from public programs but a gesture:

> I was turned down for welfare six times and then only got $10 a month. They said I had too much. I didn't have nothing but an automobile.

After a stint at the rehabilitation hospital at Warm Springs, Georgia and years of therapy, Rev. Scott was able to study accounting through a correspondence program and start a small business out of his home, and, together with his wife's income as a domestic worker, the family managed to eke out a modest living. Now, as then, Rev. Scott must budget carefully his limited funds:

> I think one has to learn to keep spending within needs, or end up with some of the needy things lacking. At first I didn't know how I would do it. There's been so many times that my little bank account was below $100. I try to spend what I get wisely. No space for throwing away anything.

None of the trials Rev. Scott endured over the years, however, was as difficult for him as the death of his wife five years ago, and he believes that only his strong faith has allowed him to overcome this loss:

> All that I had gone through was bad, but when she passed, that was harder than anything I experienced. I was so depressed, came close to committing suicide. I got a feeling I didn't have any friends, loaded up a gun, and was going to blow my brains out. I heard a voice, "Put away that gun. I'm still with you." I realized how foolish I was.

Rev. Scott now lives alone in the house he once shared with his wife. The sign out front advertising his business, "Personal Services, Taxes, Notary, Bookkeeping," is faded, and the paint is peeling badly on the outside, but inside, the house is well-maintained and, like Ms. Worth's, is neat, clean, and inviting. In the living room, where Rev. Scott still works on his accounts when he feels up to it, is a small desk, a sofa, a piano his wife used to play, a bookshelf holding mostly religious works, and, on the wall, several pictures painted by his brother. The other rooms include a kitchen, two bedrooms, and a bathroom. One bedroom Rev. Scott uses to store his accounting records; the other has his bed and television set.

Rev. Scott, himself, is neatly groomed and dressed, with signs of an increasing waistline. His grey hair and glasses give him a distinguished look. Typically reserved in manner, he becomes quite animated when explaining the various alterations (some suggested by an occupational therapist and some his own inventions) he has made in his house to accommodate his disabilities. The sofa is built up on wooden blocks, to facilitate his getting up and down, a board fitted over the bathtub enables him to bathe himself, and a plumber friend has adjusted the faucets and shower head to a height he can reach. When he lacks strength to turn the faucets, a metal pipe serves as a lever, and this same pipe helps him reach the back burners on his stove. An extra refrigerator stores staples, medicine, and housewares at a height more convenient than his kitchen cabinets; the locks on his doors turn with a handle rather than a key, easier for his arthritic hands; and the mailbox outside the front door has been lowered to wheelchair level.

Rev. Scott's house is situated on a hill, back from the street and surrounded by dilapidated, vacant houses, a night club, tall weeds, bushes, and trees. A ramp leads down from the side porch to the driveway, where his old station wagon is parked. The driveway, a mosaic of potholes, is impassable for a wheelchair, blocking his access to the street (the very one where he was struck by a car many years ago) and to the small shopping center on the other side, which houses a convenience store, barbershop, cafe, and laundromat.

Rev. Scott has lived in this house since 1953, when it was still in "the county" and had its own well and septic tank. At first he rented but was able to buy the house before his wife died. He has seen his neighborhood deteriorate over the years, and at night he often hears noises, sometimes even occasional gunshots, from the nightclub next door, the site of frequent violence. He worries that people are afraid to visit his area, and he is careful whom he lets into his home, never answering his door after dark.

## LUCY OLIVER

Lucy Oliver is seventy-five years old and has been confined to a wheelchair since suffering a stroke five years ago. She is able, with difficulty, to propel her chair and transfer from it alone, but she cannot walk and has little use of her right side. Her speech is impaired, making communication laborious and embarrassing. She is diabetic and has hypertension and mild dementia. These conditions often bring about muscle spasms and headaches and cause her to be forgetful, disoriented, anxious, and confused. As she has become more neurologically impaired, her anxiety has intensified and her cognitive abilities have diminished:

> I had a bad stroke. They told me I'd never walk again. When I gets up, I shakes all the time. My blood's [blood sugar] too high. Nothing hurts as much as [I am] just weak. I sure felt good this morning. Sometimes I feel like I'm losing my mind. I forgets things.

Mrs. Oliver lives with her husband in a one-story duplex, situated in the middle of a large (2,460 tenants) public housing project on the northwest side of town, several miles from the downtown area. Violence, usually drug-related, is common, and many units stand empty, most in a state of disrepair. The Olivers have been married for over fifty years and have lived in this same project since it was built in 1955. Here they raised their nine children, two sons and seven daughters, and one of their daughters was gunned down, caught in the cross-fire of a neighborhood skirmish.

The unit they now live in has two bedrooms, living room, kitchen, and bathroom. The small rooms are clean and tidy, but the interior has the drab institutional look typical of public housing, with concrete block walls, peeling beige paint, and linoleum floors. The focal point of the living room is a large color TV, and on the walls and sitting around on tables are pictures of their many children and grandchildren, a plant, and assorted decorative items Mrs. Oliver has brought home from the Adult Day Rehabilitation (ADR) center she attends.

The bathroom space is cramped, with barely enough room for the fixtures, a tub, and a commode with grab bars, and, as in Mrs. Washington's house, the doorway is too narrow to accommodate her wheelchair. Hence, Mrs. Oliver keeps a portable commode in her bedroom next to the double bed where she and her husband sleep. The spare room is used for storage and for their numerous cats, which multiplied from two to six during the time of this research.

When visitors come, Mrs. Oliver sits in her wheelchair or, if she is not feeling well, lies down on the sofa. She wears a housecoat and slippers. Her appearance is well-groomed, her clothes clean, and her hair neatly braided. While the television plays, she pays attention to the conversation, though is somewhat reticent because of her speech impediment.

Mrs. Oliver has lived all her life in the city. She worked for twenty-eight years as a maid in a downtown hotel while raising her family. Her husband drove a taxicab and in later years operated an informal taxi service, using his own car, until he gave up his business five years ago to care for his ailing wife.

## GERALDINE STARR

> I'm everything exceptin' dead. I don't want to give up. I'd love to
> walk again. I'm not no young woman. I'm an old woman. My heart's
> not going to take it. I have a leaking bladder. I've always had a
> leaking bladder. I'm all out of whacked. I have chronic constipation.
> I have to watch out or my bowels will break out on me. I got
> arthritis from the crown of my head to the soles of my feet. It's my
> feets and my legs. I can't stand that long. I can't lie to you. I ain't
> doing all that well. I ain't got the strength to take care of myself like
> I want to. I'm trying to tough it out. I can't get all these things on
> my mind, Miss Mary. I ain't able to think for myself.

Disabled for over two decades, the result of a stroke in 1971, Geraldine Starr, at age seventy-six, now suffers from numerous chronic conditions, physical as well as mental, including osteoarthritis, urinary dysfunction, hypertension, heart disease, anxiety, and depression. In addition, she has slight paralysis of the left side and recently had a pacemaker implanted. Over the past year she has had numerous falls. The most recent resulted in a broken hip and imposed a three-month institutionalization, initially in a hospital, then in a rehabilitation center, and, finally, three weeks in a nursing home. Back at home now, she is able to walk short distances with her walker but must use her wheelchair for most activities. She often feels overwhelmed by her many health problems.

Like Mrs. Oliver, Mrs. Starr has lived her entire life in the city. Growing up an only child, she attributes her sometimes willful ways and unsatisfying life choices to being spoiled by her mother, who had her late in life, "through the change." Although her mother was a country school teacher, Mrs. Starr dropped out of school in the eighth grade and worked in laundries or as a maid in private homes and hotels. She believes her chronic foot pain is the result of her taxing work and often laments the early choices she made:

> I've been sufferin' with my feet a good many years. I stood all day
> ironing and like to froze waitin' on the bus. Quite naturally I'm
> havin' trouble with my feets. I wish to God I had gone on and did
> better than I did, had an office. I could have been a welfare worker.
> My life is behind me now.

Mrs. Starr married for the first time when she was young, staying married "just long enough to have three sons" and then moving back home to take care of her ailing mother. She left her sons to be raised by her husband's mother, a decision she blames for their present estrangement, a source of great personal distress. Mrs. Starr married a second time a few years later, to a man she describes in similar terms to her first husband, "fine-lookin' brown-skinned man, liked good-lookin' women too," but they, too, split up, about the time her mother died in 1944. Her final marriage, although common-law and often stormy, was her most long-lasting union, over twenty years. She made the decision to leave her third husband in 1979, when he was "eaten up with cancer" and close to dying, because she could no longer tolerate his "meanness:"

> He wanted his children to help and would take it out on me when they didn't. I was lookin' for something better in the sight of God.

After separating from her third husband, Mrs. Starr moved to the large, publicly-owned and operated highrise for the elderly and handicapped where she now lives. Built in 1965, the seven-story building houses 203 mostly elderly residents in one-room efficiencies. It is located in the same neighborhood where Mrs. Starr grew up, close to the downtown area and adjacent to a lowrise project, convenience store, and rapid transit station. Because of a recent series of crimes in the public highrises, the doors to the building are kept locked, and visitors must wait to be admitted by the security guard or a passing resident and are required to sign in, stating their destination and Social Security number.

Inside the building, apartments are situated around two vast seven-story atriums, devoid of furniture and usually cold and drafty. In the front atrium, the sole decorations are an area rug and two large plants. According to Mrs. Starr, the chairs were removed because "the people [residents] couldn't keep 'em clean." Residents who wish to congregate downstairs, or even to sit to wait for rides, must do so in the community room which opens off this area. This room, where monthly meetings and occasional potluck dinners are held, is similarly uninviting with no comfortable seating area, only long tables and straight-backed chairs. The building has only two elevators, typically requiring a long wait, and the interiors of the elevators are usually dirty.

Mrs. Starr's apartment is located on the fourth floor, only about thirty feet from the elevator. She always keeps her door locked so that visitors have a lengthy wait while she makes her way slowly to the door, these days usually in her wheelchair. Inside, the one-room apartment appears cramped, with the same institutional air of the Olivers' project, but neat and clean. The front of the room serves as the living room, and contains a sofa, love seat, one table with a lamp, and a small black and white television. The rear portion of the room, where Mrs. Starr sleeps, resembles a "sick room"—the portable commode by her hospital-type bed, a small table covered with an assortment of over-the-counter remedies, liniments, and analgesics, a giant box of Depends (diaper-like pads) sitting on the floor, and her many prescription medicines lined up on the dresser. The small bathroom has a hand-icapped-accessible shower with a shower chair, an area Mrs. Starr uses to store her wash pan, mop, and bucket. A couple of plants adorn the sill of the two back windows that look out onto the small balcony, and several calendars, from years back, hang from the pegboard wall that separates the narrow kitchen area from the remainder of the room. At one end of the kitchen is a card table where Mrs. Starr eats her meals.

Although only the clutter of her furniture impedes the passage of her wheelchair, no structural changes have been made to accommodate her disability. The kitchen appliances, counters, and closets are all standard height, and the trash dump by the elevator must be operated with a foot control.

Mrs. Starr is small in stature and slightly obese. Her short, grey hair is combed straight back; her appearance is neat and clean. Like Mrs. Oliver, her usual at-home attire is a housecoat and slippers, and when visitors come, her frowning brown eyes herald the dismal conversation that inevitably will gravitate to her trials, both past and present.

## SALLY FINCH

For the past eight years, Sally Finch, aged seventy-nine, has been bound to her wheelchair by her numerous skeletal traumas—fractures of both hips, several ribs, and one knee. She also has high blood pressure and arthritis and is underweight, anemic, and anxious. Although unable either to walk or stand, she can transfer with difficulty from wheelchair to bed, shower chair, commode, or car and is able to propel herself the short distances around her apartment. Her words signify the discouragement she feels:

> There's just one thing: I wish I was able to walk. I fell against a cement wall and broke my ribs. I've been falling ever since. Walkers throw you. I have broken both hips and my knee. Oh, I've been through it. I've had back trouble since 1946—sprung spine. Gives me fits some time. If people had just told me I'd be broke up like this. . . .

Mrs. Finch migrated from the country in 1929 in search of an easier life but instead found city life to be tougher still. She started out as a maid for $5 a week and then worked in a factory for $19.20 every two weeks. During the war she operated a staple machine in a laundry. She now attributes her disabling health problems to these years of difficult labor:

> I thought I was tired of working hard, but it was worse. In the winter time you can rest [in the country]. In the city you have to work everyday. I worked, but I wasn't making anything. I mean work, from 7 A.M. to 5 P.M., thirty minutes for lunch. During war time, all day long pulling on that lever, putting on tags. At Scripto I worked the printing machine, bad on your eyes. Ain't never had no easy job. Working at private homes, didn't have no washing machine. Had to wash those clothes with your hands. Night when you go, and night when you leave.

Mrs. Finch had a long and happy marriage but has been on her own and, as she says, "catchin' hell" since her husband died in 1957. She had only one child, who died at birth, when she was seventeen years old. She was one of eight children, four boys and four girls; only she and her older sister are still living.

Like Mrs. Starr, Mrs. Finch lives alone in a federally-subsidized highrise for the elderly, where she moved five years ago when she could no longer afford the rent in her private apartment. Her building, however, is privately owned and managed and has distinct advantages over the public setting. This nine-story building is smaller (145 compared to 203 units), newer (completed in 1982), and located in a somewhat safer and less deprived area of the city, within blocks of a large private hospital and some middle-class housing. The lobby area is attractive and inviting, the community room is furnished with comfortable chairs and a large color television, and the elevators are clean and efficient. The hallways are carpeted, with handrails along the walls, and the building has a sprinkler system throughout.

The appearance of Mrs. Finch's apartment also is more appealing. She has a separate bedroom, and the rooms are spacious. The floors are carpeted, the windows—large picture windows with blinds—are clean, and the walls are freshly painted wallboard instead of concrete block. The efficiency kitchen opens into the living room where there is ample room for her daybed-style sofa, two easy chairs, a coffee table and what-not shelf, each filled with an assortment of decorations and mementos, a side table and a stand, both covered with plants. A large doll sits in one chair, and handmade pillows decorate the sofa. In the bedroom, the bed is neatly made with a bright blue bedspread. The furniture is worn and patched, but the apartment is spotlessly clean. Except for Mrs. Finch herself, little else signifies her handicapped state.

Despite the more attractive appearance of this highrise, like its public counterpart, it has few features that cater to residents in wheelchairs. The kitchen appliances and counters are standard height, as is the peephole in the front door, and the doors to the outside are not electronically controlled.

\* \* \* \* \*

With these introductions to the main characters of this book, the old people themselves, we have "set the stage" for an examination of how they experience old age, chronic disease, dependency, and the other tribulations life brings. In the following chapters, we explore in greater detail how their disabling medical conditions manifest themselves in everyday life and the impact that disease and disability have on their abilities to live independently. It is already clear that a wide range of frailties exist—from Mrs. Little, who is bedridden, to Ms. Worth, who can get about on her walker. They differ also in how they view their health statuses—Rev. Scott does not "feel sick," yet Mrs. Little considers herself "half-dead," while Mrs. Starr is "everything exceptin' dead."

Lifetimes of perseverance, self-reliance, and hard work have contributed to the many strengths these seven African American elders manifest as they continue their struggle to cope with their failing capacities. Critical to this struggle is preserving, as best they can, their independence. A recurring theme throughout this book is the ideal of independence juxtaposed against the reality of dependence. While the realization that help is needed is ever-present, each person strives to avoid the trials of dependency. We will see great variation in the degree to which this goal is achieved. What these differences mean in the lives of these poor, old, black, and impaired persons, and to their needs for and uses of long-term care is the focus of this book.

## REFERENCES

1. E. Goffman, *The Presentation of Self in Everyday Life*, Anchor Books, New York, 1959.
2. R. L. Rubinstein, J. C. Kilbride, and S. Nagy, *Elders Living Alone*, Aldine de Gruyter, New York, 1992.

3. S. Matthews, *The Social World of Old Women: Management of Self-Identity*, Sage Publications Inc., Beverly Hills, California, 1979.
4. M. P. Lawton and L. Nahemow, Ecology and the Aging Process, in *The Psychology of Adult Development and Aging*, C. Eisdorfer and M. P. Lawton (eds.), American Psychological Association, Washington, D. C., pp. 619-674, 1973.

# CHAPTER
2

# Abilities and Disabilities

*So many things are hard for me.*
Rev. Scott

Sometimes it seems to Geraldine Starr that her body is under attack, and sometimes she feels like jolts of electricity are shooting through her feet. This pain she suffers as a result of her arthritis is debilitating and depressing. Her words are graphic and poignant:

> I aches all over, all across my shoulders, just like somebody stabbin' me with a knife. My legs is painin' me so bad. Arthritis goes 'way down in my foot and spreads like electricity. I can't do like I want to do. It's too much trouble. That's the reason I didn't fix me nothing to eat yet. I couldn't stand up. My legs are sore as a boil. That's what tears me up—walking to the refrigerator, back to the table, gives me all those pains. I try to stay off my feet and keep this swelling down. They swelling so bad, by the time I get my feet out of that bed and put them down and walk from here to the TV and from there to the bathroom, they done popped up that quick. They stay down as long as I'm off of them because there's no pressure on them, but time I get up and start to walking, they pop right back up. Sometimes they look like they're going to bust. I can't empty the garbage; I can't go to the mailbox; I can't go down and pay my rent. I'm just settin' here like I'm in a hole, like I can't get out. I can't do nothing for myself. *That's* what's killing me. Sometimes I wouldn't care if I just die and get it over with. It's a struggle to stay here in life. I don't want to be where I can't help myself. It's almost more than I can bear sometime. My nerves is so bad. I goes all to pieces. I've never been that way. My pains and things works on my mind. This is the worsest pains that I've ever been in. I'm tired of painin'. I go to the edge. I don't want to commit suicide, but I sure feel like it.

When Mrs. Starr's depressive symptoms appear in all their force, her functional abilities are further limited, thus creating a circular chain of events.

As this brief moment from Geraldine Starr's daily struggle with life illustrates, her chief concern is not with whatever medical diagnoses may have been noted in her case records but with how she feels when she gets up in the morning and how those feelings can interfere with her daily activities. As many have noted, such issues are also the central focus of long-term care, and especially home care. Not the disease but the dysfunction is paramount. The ability to manage independently, to carry out the necessary tasks of daily life, is all that many people ask of their old age.

Among these seven African American elders, a considerable variability exists in their ability to perform these tasks. Still the words of Rev. Scott at the beginning of this chapter could have come from any one of them. All activities require more effort and take more time than if they were carried out by an unimpaired person. This rather obvious fact influences the increased importance often attached to routine activities by disabled persons and affects their ability to be independent. Just getting up, bathed, dressed, and fed can consume an entire day and expend one's store of energy. Yet, as Mrs. Starr expresses, performing the most routine activity independently often brings great satisfaction:

When I get up, I feel like I've accomplished something.

Despite numerous barriers and hardships, many personal care tasks (Activities of Daily Living—ADL's) and even homemaking activities (Instrumental Activities of Daily Living—IADL's) still can be carried out independently by these old people—even those with significant disabilities. All, however, need at least partial help with some of these chores. No one can do any heavy cleaning, get out of the house on their own, do regular cooking, or even completely bathe and dress unassisted. In keeping with previous research [1], we found the problems encountered in performing these routine activities related to the physical demands of the task.

We also discovered, as many others have, that disability is a complex and multidimensional phenomenon. Schulz and Williamson developed a conceptual model to help explain the impact of disabling conditions on the physical and psychological morbidity and the quality of life of patients and their family members [2]. This model follows the framework of traditional stress-coping models and is based on the assumption that both the psychological representations of illness and disability and the social contexts in which they occur are significant determinants of the impact of physical frailty. Four essential elements of the model are identified: the objective conditions that cause the stress, the perception of stress, the lasting outcomes of the stress, and various conditioning or situational variables that can moderate the relationships between stressors and their impact on patients and their families.

We noted many similarities in the factors that affect the daily lives of these participants. The magnitude of their disabilities and the symptoms associated with their chronic conditions clearly influence their distress levels and depressive symptomology, and the negative outcomes of stress are greater when the disabling conditions interfere with their normal activities.

Schulz and Williamson found prognosis of the condition and length of time since onset influenced the outcomes of stress [2]. We too learned that while the permanence of chronic disease contributes to its difficulty, the years spent living with disability can facilitate coping. Schulz and Williamson identified additional factors that act as intervening variables, moderating the relationship between stressors and the impact on the patient [2]. We noted similar situational factors, such as gender, income, social support, personality, and coping strategies used, affecting the outcomes of disability.

DeFriese and colleagues offer additional insight from the self-care literature [3]. They discuss three dimensions of self-care that people with chronic health problems practice in response to their functional limitations: 1) use of special equipment and assistive technology; 2) physical changes in the environment; and 3) behavioral adjustments in daily activities. These authors note, as we have, that self-care is not carried out in an environmental vacuum but within a socio-cultural context. How individuals respond to the disability—the practices they adopt—is influenced by such factors as social support, socioeconomic status, motivation, and personal skills and resources for self-care. These factors influence their capacities to maintain a balance between the challenges of their environments—that is, environmental press [4]—and their competence in managing their daily lives.

The concept of self-care is not new to our informants, and the degree of independence each of these seven elders is able to achieve in performing tasks of daily living depends on the complete array of each person's remaining resources—intellectual, physical, material, social, psychological, and spiritual. These elders often adjust their behavior in the practice of self-care, and it is the distribution of resources among these categories that determines the strategies they use to perform activities basic to life. Although all categories of resources are significant for creating personal strategies, when physical, intellectual, material, and social resources fail, often it is the strategies dependent on psychological and spiritual resources that help people pull through. It is these categories of resources that permit individuals faced with the realities of chronic disease and disability greater success in adapting to their circumstances. The ability to adapt enables them to maximize their remaining resources.

Often in these situations adaptation means the capacity to focus on, and derive satisfaction from, the abilities that one still has rather than on the more obvious deficiencies or, simply, "to make the best of a bad situation." Rubinstein and colleagues described analogous behavior among a group of similarly impaired elders [5]. By a process called the *"miniaturization of satisfaction,"* people for whom few possibilities remain in life base their decisions about satisfaction in the realm of small, rather than large, events. Thus, Geraldine Starr, who once loved to get out of her house and "just go," is happier when she can accept her impaired condition (which she cannot always do), deriving satisfaction from her more scaled-down accomplishments, such as being able to get out of her bed each day. Through acceptance of her restricted options, Viola Worth can be happy with what she *can* do and not be unduly distraught over what she cannot. In many ways these African American elders resemble Myerhoff's Jewish old people, who derived similar satisfactions from managing the small chores of daily life, often against incredible odds [6]. In Myerhoff's words, these accomplishments, "should be counted as successful examples of the lifework of aging" [6, p. 252].

Although most of these participants are able to adapt psychologically to their conditions, few have made physical or social changes in their environments because of their increased impairments. Only minimal design changes have been made to the interiors and exteriors of their homes, and no one is considering future changes in their living arrangements. Many environmental changes would be prohibited because of inadequate finances, yet little interest in making such changes was even expressed by these individuals. Each person, however, did use some type of assistive device at times, often of their own devising.

Wister found similar coping strategies among incapacitated old people in Canada [7]. The findings from his study, which assessed Lawton and Nahemow's ecological model of aging, depicted these elders as people who engaged in psychological adaptation to their home environments rather than altering the physical and social characteristics [4]. Like the seven elders in our book, these Canadian elders gradually accepted a variety of health-related inconveniences and developed innovative strategies to negotiate an increasingly demanding environment.

DeFriese and colleagues report on a recent national survey of self-care practices among a national probability sample of persons over age sixty-five [3]. The results of this study show again that older persons are far more likely to chose behavioral modification over changing the environment or using special equipment to compensate for disability.

In this chapter we will examine the abilities of these individuals to carry out basic tasks of everyday living, including those relating to personal care (ADL) and those having to do with household management (IADL). It is clear that each success—each ability maintained for another day—is both hard-won and highly valued by its author, a personal claim staked to independence and identity.

## PERSONAL CARE TASKS

Personal care activities, including bowel and bladder functions, personal hygiene, and dressing, are an essential part of each day. Bowel and bladder activities cause significant problems for several of these elders, particularly those who, in addition to their limited mobility, experience frequent urination or incontinence. For them, toileting often requires the use of various preparations and paraphernalia, including portable bedside commodes, bedpans, disposable diapers, protective pads for bedding, urinary catheters, and certain medications.

Geraldine Starr uses a bedside commode and puts newspapers and pads on her bed at night. During the day she wears diaper-like pads. She can manage these tasks alone, but considerable effort is required to empty the commode, using either her wheelchair or walker, even though distances are short in her one-room efficiency apartment. Since she has difficulty standing, changing her urinary pads is a lengthy and precarious process. Most mornings she has soaked through her night clothes and pads, and twice during the past year she has fallen while getting up to urinate during the night, once turning over the portable commode, unable on both occasions to rise from the floor by herself. Her words vividly describe her nocturnal trials:

> My pee's drivin' me crazy. My pee leaks out of me. I'm soaking wet. When I wake up, I be in a puddle of pee. I don't know where that pee comes from. I generally don't sleep. I tend to stay woke all night. More than likely I'm going to have to urinate; then I have to wash my hands, empty the water out, and put some clean water in. Sometimes I sit down on the commode and I just set there. Even if

> I close my eyes, I don't go to sleep much. Then I'll sort of doze off, but I'll wake up and say, "Lord, let me get out of this bathroom." I have to pee so regular, and when I wake up in my sleep, I'm so way out, I can't get myself together. I sit down there and I be done urinated and I'm still sleep. Don't wake up good. That's the reason I fell. I don't know how I fell out that bed. I woke up and I was lying on my face.

Ruby Washington's comparable problems are exacerbated by her diabetic condition:

> I have to go a whole lot of times with sugar [diabetes], every hour when my sugar actin' up. When you have diabetes you takes more leaks.

Because her wheelchair cannot fit into her bathroom, she routinely uses a bedpan or portable commode, both of which require the help of another person. Sometimes at night, she does not wake up in time, compounding her personal hygiene problems:

> I just have to do like I do in the hospital, just get my pee can. Jack [a neighborhood helper] always carries my wet out. I gets up two or three times at night and take a leak. I sit on the side of the bed and slide. If I be in a hurry, I get my pan. I be asleep sometimes and have to go. I can't tell. I wakes up and be wet. If I wet the bed, I have to change everyday. I got a rubber sheet I put under the sheet.

Viola Worth, too, has particular problems at night with frequent urination. She explains how these aggravating symptoms routinely interfere with her rest:

> It's a mess. I have the stool as close to bed as I can get it. I have to jump up and down so regular. By the time I get comfortable, I have to get up and pee. Last night I went to sleep for thirty minutes, headed to the stool. I can make it about an hour and a half.

Eloise Little is no longer able to tend to any bowel or bladder tasks independently. Unable to get out of bed unassisted, she must use diapers and a urinary catheter and lay in bed till someone can help her. When she still was able to make it on her own from her bed to the bedside commode, it was a tedious and long-drawn out process, requiring about five minutes each way, but she always insisted on doing it by herself and found "moving slow" to be her best strategy:

> I moves slow, but I makes it. I have to take my time. I fell so much.

Because this undertaking was so laborious, Mrs. Little often stayed on the commode for long periods of time. From her bedside seat, she used her "special wire" carefully to arrange the pads and paper bags that protected her bed.

Personal hygiene, such as bathing, hair washing, and nail cutting, also is difficult for these people to manage, and these tasks become more onerous with conditions such as incontinence and lack of bowel control. No one can do any of these tasks quickly or easily, and in most cases, an essential part of the process requires assistance. Ruby Washington is able to give herself a bed bath if someone brings her the necessary items; to dress and comb her hair, but not wash it; and to cut her fingernails on the left hand, but not the right. Viola Worth needs help getting in and out of her old-fashioned tub and washing her back, and Sally Finch, although able to transfer from her wheelchair to the shower chair, cannot operate the handheld shower.

Personal strategies have been developed to enhance independence. Geraldine Starr, who must wash off every morning when she first gets up because of her frequent incontinence at night, only takes a "good bath" once or twice a week. She manages best washing herself by hand, instead of in the shower, but she still finds the procedure arduous and frustrating and compares herself to a helpless baby:

> I do good with my bath. I gets a dry wash cloth and holds on to the sink and the shower door. I can rinse the soap out of my skin real good, but it's complicated washing my back. I have to get a towel. I can't use my left arm to wash my right arm. That's the hell of it. I'm just like a newborn baby.

Sometimes, because of fluctuations in her condition, Mrs. Starr is not able to accomplish this task at all:

> I can clean myself up sometimes, and sometimes I can't. I goes and comes. Sometimes I'm stronger than others, sometimes I'm weaker than others.

Others also have devised strategies to facilitate their independent care. Ms. Worth's gheri-curls (a type of permanent wave) enable her to comb and style her own hair with greater ease, and Rev. Scott uses a number of mechanical devices for self-care, such as his specially designed shower fixtures and board for bathing and two unique homemade gadgets—a pair of fingernail clippers affixed to a board and a comb with an extended handle. Still, limited mobility prevents his washing his own hair or feet.

Putting on clothes can be a frustrating, difficult, and even dangerous task for individuals who are weak, unsteady, and have limited use of their hands. Mrs. Starr fell and broke her hip while getting undressed after a tiring day of medical tests. Yet, with the exception of Mrs. Little, each of these old people, given enough time, is able to manage at least most of this activity alone, and each has devised ways of facilitating the process.

Rev. Scott uses a button hook for buttoning his shirts, and Mrs. Finch, whose limited mobility is compounded by her nervous condition, allows herself plenty of time. Sometimes Mrs. Finch's strategy is not to get dressed at all, an acceptable option for her because she has few social interactions. Her description of her anxiety is telling:

> I have the hardest trouble getting dressed. If I gets in a hurry, I get nervous and can't do nothing. I be wondering if this be right, that be right. When I'm going to the doctor, I get my clothes together a day ahead of time. I needs plenty of time to do things. If I try to hurry I be trembling, drop things. Sometimes I keep my pajamas on all day. Sometimes I just feel like putting something on. I put my clothes on yesterday, thinking somebody coming. Nobody came. Sometimes I don't feel like it.

Always fearful of falling, as she has done numerous times, Mrs. Starr dresses sitting down:

> I have to sit down when I put my clothes on. I just don't want to fall no more.

And she wears house shoes around her apartment to accommodate her incontinence:

> When my water starts coming, I have to slip out of them. I hate to wet my shoes.

She and Lucy Oliver both keep their house coats on during the day to facilitate frequent trips to the bathroom. Similarly, Ms. Worth wears pants with elastic waistbands. Unable to dress herself at all, Mrs. Little always wears her nightgown, even when going to the clinic.

## HOUSEHOLD TASKS

As with personal care tasks, there is a wide range in the abilities of this group of impaired elders to perform household tasks, yet no one is able to do all needed chores unassisted. Again, the capability to manage care independently depends on each person's physical and mental states and on the availability of certain equipment or a helper to furnish an intermediary service.

Abilities often are based on past experiences. For the women in this group, many of the instrumental tasks of daily living were a regular part of both their personal and their professional lives, and their past successes now help them cope with their present trials. Although Rev. Scott is unaccustomed to performing the housekeeping chores that were once his wife's sole domain, his accounting experiences serve him well.

Taking care of personal business, especially managing one's money is the instrumental task that each of these individuals finds most salient and, thus, strives hardest to preserve. Even Mrs. Little takes charge of her finances, though not always with competence. She keeps her money and her important papers within her reach at all times—her "main" money stays pinned to her nightgown, inside her "brother-in-law sack" (a little bag given to her by this person), and her "nickel and dime bank" is two snuff cans, one inside the other. Another little barrel holds her pennies, to pay her bills if she does not have "cash money." Although usually adept at doling her money out, she sometimes loses track of where it goes or loses it altogether. Still she remains resolute in her resistance to her family's control:

> Everybody don't have an idea what to do with money. *I* do. Gertrude thinks I drink it up. I don't need nobody to inch it out to me. I ain't quite lost my mind yet.

The other participants, with the exception of Mrs. Oliver, whose cognitive deficits limit her abilities, have no difficulty managing their money but do need help paying bills or getting checks cashed. For most, inexperience in the business world prevents the use of commercial banks and the paying of bills by mail. Only Mrs. Oliver and Rev. Scott have checking accounts, and bill paying for the others necessitates trips to utility companies or the purchase of money orders, both requiring assistance.

Other business matters frequently entail dealing with the various government agencies that provide assistance, and these older people usually must have help in reading, interpreting, and filling out the necessary forms, an area where the first author was able to provide assistance.

The difficulties associated with business tasks are for some related to lack of education as well as to physical and mental disabilities. Only

Mrs. Washington has visual problems severe enough to interfere with reading, but Mrs. Oliver's right side impairment, as well as her fluctuating cognitive skills, hinder her ability to write and to comprehend procedures. For Sally Finch, the impact on her right hand of many years operating a staple machine impedes her writing abilities. Ms. Worth lacks reading skills, and Mrs. Starr's mental problems frequently handicap her proficiency, often causing her to become quite agitated when dealing with representatives of various institutions or looking for necessary papers:

> My nerves are just bad since I had my stroke. If I be talking to her, I be done blowed my top. . . . She got me in such a tumble, I didn't know which a way I was going. The harder I looked, the further away it [a needed document] got.

Each person needs help with shopping since no one is still able to drive a car or ride the bus, although all but Mrs. Little could manage portions of this chore if they had transportation and some assistance. When Viola Worth can locate someone to take her to a grocery store, which she often can, she gets particular satisfaction out of pushing the cart around the store herself and making her own selections. At one time Lucy Oliver's husband regularly pushed her in her wheelchair to the neighborhood market, allowing her at least to direct the shopping, but when guard rails were installed at the public entrance to prevent cart theft, the accessibility of Mrs. Oliver's wheelchair also was denied. Geraldine Starr chooses to have her groceries delivered from a nearby market, despite many complaints about the poor quality and high prices.

Each of these persons also requires at least partial assistance with other routine housekeeping chores, such as cooking, cleaning, and washing. Mrs. Little and Mrs. Washington need complete care in these areas, and Mrs. Oliver's limited mobility allows her, with great difficulty, only to make her bed and dust. The four individuals who are somewhat less disabled can manage a number of household tasks, when they have the necessary time and energy and when they are motivated to put forth the extra effort that is always required. It takes Rev. Scott, for example, an hour and a half to prepare and eat his breakfast and Mrs. Finch, a half an hour to make her bed:

> Takes half hour to make the bed, half hour to bathe, an hour to put on my clothes, when I put on some. Then I have to fix breakfast, such as it is. Sometimes I don't have anything but toast and coffee.

Time, for these older persons, is a resource that is valuable and, thankfully, usually plentiful. A good portion of each day can be spent just taking care of these basic needs.

As with personal care tasks, these elders have developed strategies that enable them to use their remaining resources to best advantage. The use of assistive devices again enhances the independence of some informants. Rev. Scott, true to his pattern of using tools, employs a long stick to make his bed and a commercial claw-like device he calls his "reacher" to facilitate a variety of chores, such as opening the latch on the screen door or carrying items in a plastic bag from the refrigerator to the counter. For Mrs. Finch, a cut-off broom enables her to sweep the carpet while seated in her wheelchair. Geraldine Starr, on the other hand, resists change and scorns the assistive devices she acquired while in the rehabilitation hospital.

Others discover new ways of doing old chores. Viola Worth has changed her way of cooking, now baking things in the oven, rather than frying them on top of the stove, a process which required long periods of standing. She has even learned to use her microwave, a device she resisted at first as "too new-fangled." Another strategy of Ms. Worth's is to use her chair, rather than her walker, when she does chores she finds difficult or particularly time-consuming, for example, putting away her groceries. She paces herself and is quite pleased with her accomplishments:

> I learn ways about different things. I hold on to things, catch to the stove, hold to the table. I don't try to do too much. If I want some bacon, I put it in a container, put the oven on, and go about my business. I don't have fried food too much because I don't feel like standing there tending to it, and I have learned to put my stuff in the stove, and I like it better that way. I can't stand that good, and I'm so proud that I can do as well as I do.

For these frail elders, being able to adjust to their greatly reduced capacities enables them to maximize their independence, for all a positive achievement. It is often the pleasure derived from this independence, even when extraordinary effort is required, that is the motivating force. The satisfaction Mrs. Starr gets from performing tasks herself motivates her to put forth the extra effort and sometimes even lessens the symptoms of disease:

> I like to do my own cooking. I feel better when I'm in the kitchen cooking or in that bathroom working. I lay in bed and think of a thousand things to do. I get weak as water, and I lie down till my

strength comes back. Then I get up again. I'm more happier when I'm doing something. I want to be doing something, but I ain't able to do the things I want to do. I can't [just] look at my hands.

For Mrs. Finch, too, keeping house helps to relieve her frequent boredom and improve her mental health. Comparing herself to a fox, she makes an effort to emphasize the value of these pursuits:

I do what I can. I'm like a fox. You know a fox will keep a clean place. There's always something to do around the house. That's what I do to keep my mind together, keep from sitting here looking at the walls.

As with ADL tasks, the ability to carry out IADL tasks independently (and the burden of a particular task) varies with fluctuations in the symptoms of disease. Pain, a common complaint of each of these participants, is capricious in its assault and thus its impact on independent care. The response of individuals to pain and the ability to manage it is variable as well. As we noted at the beginning of this chapter, when Mrs. Starr is in extreme pain, her self-care activities are curtailed and her depression becomes more severe. Ms. Worth's pain is not as regular or severe, though she still has her bad days, nor does she allow her pain to impede her activities in the way that Mrs. Starr does:

I'm still draggin'. My hip is extra stiff. I be stiff, but I'm not in no real pain. I just don't know. Everybody have those days. It ain't hurtin' that bad 'cause I'm still doing the twist [the dance of the sixties]. I think I'll be all right. I get tired sometimes if it always look like I'm complainin'. I don't tell nobody all the time how I be feeling. I just keep a goin'.

Certain factors related to the environment or to the material resources of these elders also act to promote or inhibit further independence in performing IADL activities. Because Ms. Worth owns a washing machine and a freezer, she can do her own laundry and buy her groceries in bulk. On the other hand, none of the homeowners is financially able to create a barrier-free or completely accessible environment within their homes or to have barrier-free access to the outdoors. All persons live in unsafe areas or areas that lack convenient, reasonably priced, high quality services.

When the needs of these older persons are particularly great or when tasks require special effort, they draw on their psychological and spiritual resources in their struggle to cope with daily life. Viola Worth, for one, attributes many of the successes she has to her will to keep trying:

> I don't grieve. I just try. I'm not going to give up. As long as I can scuffle, I'm gonna scuffle. I'll leave here quicker [die] if I have help. I'm so proud that I can do as well as I do. As long as you got the will power, I feel you'll make it somehow. If you give up and say, "I can't," you just can't. I'm still trying. If I give up, I'll be sittin' up here like a folded-up something or other.

In her view, this strength ultimately is derived from the "power of God," a belief shared by each of these older African Americans:

> I travel by faith. Life is faith. If you don't have faith you're gonna live, you ain't gonna live. If I ain't got faith, I'm not gonna be able to get up from here and go back to that bathroom. My faith is what keepin' me going. I was raised here with God, and I know there's something or other that talks to me beside humans. That little voice I hear. That's what helps me a lot. I talk to the spirit of God just like I talk to you and ask him to take care of me. I say, "Lord, I know I have a hard way," and before I know anything, I've done it myself.

Not everyone has the faith and inner fortitude—the spiritual and psychological resources—necessary to motivate them to ever greater levels of endeavor. Some people succumb to the trials of the battle, maybe just for a day or two, but the threat of permanent surrender is always present. Geraldine Starr's response to her situation illustrates how disease and disability can take its toll. When her myriad of symptoms act in unison, she reaches the brink of her endurance:

> I done lived my life. If you're dead, all your troubles are over with. I wish I could just die in peace, breathe my last. I ain't hardly going to be able to do anything else, just walk around half dead. I want to go on living; then I don't want to live. I ask the Lord, "What am I living for?" I ain't got no more value. Since I' been sick like this, I get all mixed up. I hadn't been like that. Too much stress on me, I can't map it out, worrying about my sickness. I know I'll never get well. I ain't feeling too good now, peculiar feeling in my neck. I don't know what to do. Varicose veins feel like they about to bust. It scares me sometime. Been having terrible pains in my stomach. I hope it's not cancer. Doctor said it could go into it. Lord, what must I do? What's going to become of me? Life gets so complicated. I don't want to suffer. I'd rather be dead. But you can't commit suicide—

would go straight to hell. If I could just close my eyes without killing myself, I would be so happy.

\* \* \* \* \*

Despite the toll disease and disability have taken on the reality of independence for each of these survivors, the ideal is still strong. The desire to take care of their own needs is rooted firmly in the value of independence and in their abhorrence of dependency—concepts we explore further in Chapters 6 and 7. Their resolve to perform a task independently is affected as well by the availability of help from others and by their attitude toward that help. If no one else is available to do a needed task, or if a helper's performance is unacceptable, an individual sometimes will try a little harder for self-reliance.

## REFERENCES

1. S. J. Czaja, R. A. Weber, and S. N. Nair, A Human Factor Analysis of ADL Activities: A Capability Demand Approach, *Journal of Gerontology, 48*, pp. 44-50, 1993.
2. R. Schulz and G. M. Williamson, Psychosocial and Behavioral Dimensions of Physical Frailty, *Journal of Gerontology, 48*, Supplement, pp. 39-43, 1993.
3. G. H. DeFriese, T. R. Konrad, A. Woomert, J. K. Norburn, and S. Bernard, Self-Care and Quality of Life in Old Age, in *Aging and Quality of Life: Charting New Territories in Behavioral Science Research*, R. P. Abeles, H. G. Gift, and M. G. Ory (eds.), Springer Publishing Company, New York, pp. 99-117, 1994.
4. M. P. Lawton and L. Nahemow, Ecology and the Aging Process, in *The Psychology of Adult Development and Aging*, C. Eisdorfer and M. P. Lawton (eds.), American Psychological Association, Washington, D. C., pp. 619-674, 1973.
5. R. L. Rubinstein, B. B. Alexander, M. Goodman, and M. Luborsky, Key Relationships of Never Married, Childless Older Women: A Cultural Analysis, *Journal of Gerontology: Social Sciences, 46*:5, pp. S270-S277, 1991.
6. B. Myerhoff, *Number Our Days*, Simon & Schuster, New York, 1978.
7. A. V. Wister, Environmental Adaptation by Persons in Their Later Life, *Research on Aging, 11*:3, pp. 267-291, 1989.

# CHAPTER
# 3

# Health Care Practices

*It's a pity what these doctors do to old people.*
Geraldine Starr

It is 5 P.M. Sally Finch sits alone in her wheelchair, hungry, thirsty, exhausted, and ignored. She has come to County Hospital for help but may well end the day in worse shape than when she left home at 8:00 A.M. this morning. Despite her age and disability, she has come alone, as she often does, to the outpatient clinic at County, seeking relief from her ailments within the system of poverty medicine that is supposed to care for her. Today, however, she has been defeated in her quest. She is as much a victim of the system as of her failing body.

It is hard to describe just how difficult it sometimes is for poor, elderly people to obtain health care. While illness and disability are the central facts of everyday life for these seven black older persons, other factors—such as poverty, lack of education, and a lifetime of difficulties with powerful bureaucracies—help to define what kind of sick people they are and what kind of care they receive.

A crucial but often-overlooked part of the long-term care system is its intersection with the acute health care system. Chronically ill patients, even those who require extensive supportive care best delivered at home, find they often must journey to acute care settings to submit themselves to physicians or other professionals. Less often, but with more negative effect, these long-term care clients must be hospitalized for treatment of acute conditions or acute episodes of existing chronic diseases. The net effect is that doctors and acute care nurses, who have little formal specialized training in geriatrics and usually even less in the unique problems of the poor, are often ill-equipped to provide appropriate, high quality care to the elderly poor, or to articulate their care with that of the long-term care system.

53

On the other hand, the values, attitudes, and social networks of older patients strongly influence the kind of care they want and need and, to some extent, the kind they receive. As Twaddle and Hessler have pointed out, being sick is at once a physical, a psychological, and a social phenomenon [1]. The physical dimension, termed by these authors "disease," is recognized by its characteristics, or "signs," that can be measured objectively and so do not depend on the individual's perceptions. While physicians are primarily concerned with diagnosing disease—naming and classifying a collection of scientifically measured signs and patient-reported feelings, or symptoms, patients also seek to "name" their conditions in order to classify and understand them. Most people, including our participants, largely accept the dominant medical-scientific model, even if they don't understand how it works. Some, including some of these older African Americans, also subscribe to competing theories of disease cause and cure, including divine intervention and fate.

"Illness" is the psychological manifestation usually recognized first by the individual who experiences "symptoms," or subjective feelings of not being well that are judged important and likely to interfere with the ability to function. Common symptoms include pain, dizziness, and nausea, feelings not apparent to others or susceptible to objective measurement. Symptoms may or may not be indicators of disease, but they almost always create concern in the individual experiencing them and generally lead to some effort to treat them. Individuals tend to define their problems in terms of illness, while practitioners think primarily in terms of disease. The participants in our study were no exception, referring in conversation primarily to their feelings rather than their disease.

The third dimension of nonhealth is "sickness," the social identity of sick person that must be defined by others. Sickness is usually defined as the inability to function in one's normal activities. By legitimating non-performance of normal roles, it accords the person protection from a deviant label. In return it demands a therapeutic response on the part of the sick person. The participants we observed have little trouble being defined as sick in order to receive both formal and informal support and forbearance. Nor do they have a problem in accepting the legitimation conferred by their conditions. Most occasionally fail to fulfill their therapeutic obligations of seeking help, keeping appointments at the clinic, or following the doctor's instructions (e.g., in taking their medications). Ness has explained the difficulty inherent in the sick role for someone who has a chronic condition, which offers no hope of recovery [2]. In such cases the role of sick person must be integrated with one's preferred normal roles if identity and self-esteem are to be retained. While such an integrated set of roles was difficult for all, and quite impossible for some, none of these people seemed to have any trouble maintaining their legitimacy as "sick people." This was probably because the objective reality of disease and frailty was so apparent and because the formal care system has no incentive to enforce these unwritten rules of sickness.

Although all three dimensions may be present and recognized in an individual, one or the other tends to be emphasized, depending on whose point of view is considered. Physicians tend to focus on disease, with its accompanying signs of physical dysfunction, while the patient may dwell more on his or her subjective feelings of illness or how the condition interferes with normal social roles.

It is also true that individuals with similar health conditions and degree of impairment often experience them differently and, in fact, may behave in quite different ways. Illness behavior, according to Mechanic, is the way in which a person perceives, evaluates, and acts upon the manifestations of illness (disease) [3]. Despite their many common problems, these seven individuals clearly differ in the way they perceive their ailments, in how they evaluate the meaning of these ailments for their lives, and in what they chose to do about them. Some feel the burden of their conditions very acutely, while others, objectively just as impaired, minimize their symptoms. Some appear to accept their conditions impassively, while others still hope to get better. Some are active in their search for help and cooperative with caregivers; others assume help to be unavailable, ineffective, or incompatible with their needs and consistently fail to comply with medical instructions.

In this chapter we examine the medical self-care practices of these seven old people in the context of the long-term care system available to them. Our focus is on their use of physicians and acute health care facilities, how they perceive the services received, and how they act, or fail to act, upon the advice and directives of their health care providers. In each case, we identify factors—both in the individual and in the system—that influence their illness behaviors, paying particular attention to those that act as barriers to good health care practices.

## UTILIZATION OF ACUTE CARE SERVICES

### Going to the Doctor

Each of these individuals regularly visits a doctor who monitors her or his conditions and recommends various therapeutic regimens. These physicians are either in private practice or based at the large public hospital, County Memorial, located downtown and designed to serve the indigent. Because of their limited incomes, each qualifies for Medicaid, as well as Medicare, and, through these two programs, most in- and out-patient services, prescribed medications and treatments, and transportation to medically-related appointments may be obtained free of charge. Unfortunately, the reluctance of many physicians in private practice to accept patients without private medical insurance often means that poor people have little choice but to use public facilities.

Although Geraldine Starr was born at "black" County, as it was called in the days before desegregation, and Viola Worth still calls County her "home," they now shun the public hospital and use only private physicians. Joseph Scott makes regular visits to the rheumatology and cardiology clinics at County, but private vascular and plastic surgeons take care of his leg ulcers and skin grafts. The other four individuals continue, as they always have, to use only the public hospital, regularly attending County's outpatient clinics for their primary care. This distinction between private and public care is significant, in terms both of the quality of care received and of the need for assistance in utilizing medical services.

The use of the large public clinics at County entails many difficulties, particularly for someone who is mentally or physically impaired and possibly alone. One problem is County's immense size, with long corridors, slow elevators, and over-crowded clinics typically requiring endless waits. A recent visit for Eloise Little to the medical clinic lasted four hours, including the wait for the medical transportation service. If a patient is alone, problems are compounded, since no one is present to advocate for the patient, who is often unwilling, or unable, to be assertive. When Mrs. Little is by herself, she waits silently in her wheelchair, or on a stretcher, until someone notices her, oftentimes after all the other patients have gone home. A stop by the hospital pharmacy to get medicine incurs an additional wait. Mrs. Finch's sentiments are representative:

> I stayed over there till 5 o'clock, no water, nothing to eat. It was pretty rough. I had to wait so long, just wore me out. I was tired, tired. Can't go anywhere else. They charge too much.

Mrs. Finch believes she has no other options for medical care because she is poor. Unlike those who have abandoned County, she has neither the knowledge nor the skills herself, nor a capable helper, to find a private physician willing to accept her as a Medicaid patient.

Other difficulties, especially for wheelchair-bound patients, involve routine clinic procedures that require patients to maneuver through narrow hallways and go to other floors to be weighed, give a urine specimen, have blood drawn, get medications, or make future appointments. At Mrs. Finch's regular appointment at the medical clinic, located on the second floor, she was asked to go to the radiology department on the third floor and to the gynecology department on the fifth floor to make appointments for additional tests. On this particular day, the first author had accompanied Mrs. Finch and made these trips for her, but had Mrs. Finch been alone, as she often is, she simply would have ignored these requests. This day she made no attempt to go to the pharmacy located on the ground floor to get the medicine prescribed by the doctor, choosing, as she does routinely, to pay someone to pick it up for her another day. Mrs. Finch's graphic words illustrate the difficulties she experiences on a typical visit to County, in her wheelchair and alone:

> When you get to the hospital, they don't have people to help you. I put my appointment in the door. Then I got to go back around to sign my name. If somebody with me, they can go for me. They wanted me to go on the third floor to take a flu shot, but I told 'em I couldn't go. I need someone to push me around. It's terrible. Sometimes they want your urine. I can't go to the bathroom to get urine by myself. If I go downstairs to get my medicine, you know the line always be from the door all the way around. Nobody's gonna let you in front of them, I don't care what shape you're in.

Rev. Scott, who always makes his clinic visits by himself, encounters similar problems and on occasion even has to cross the street to get to the lab in another building. Now that he has a power chair, he has little difficulty navigating the interior of the building, but he once found such travel exhausting and still is fearful of crossing the street:

> Before I was given the power chair, it was trouble trying to push my chair up the halls. It was more than I could do. Sometimes someone would give me a little push. . . . I don't fancy the idea of getting out on the street by myself.

Sometimes wheelchair patients are the last to see the doctor. On one visit Mrs. Little was the last patient to leave the medical clinic, and Mr. Oliver related how his wife routinely endures similar discrimination:

> They make them [people in wheelchairs] sit outside and wait till everyone gets waited on. They call you, "Oh, you in a wheelchair. We'll get you after awhile." You know that's true. What difference does it make? They're not slow about sending the bill!

Additional problems concern the physician, typically a physician in training (a resident), and the actual examination. Physician turnover is high, preventing any long-term continuity of care or familiarity with the patient or the patient's condition and limiting development of rapport. None of these County patients could identify by name a doctor who had treated them. Additionally, the majority of County physicians are young, white, and middle-class, with little practical knowledge of home care needs or experience in dealing with older patients with chronic problems. Together with the obvious cultural differences, these experience deficits contribute to a lack of communication and understanding. The white male resident who examined Mrs. Little had no awareness of her need for diapers or protective bed pads, and had the first author not been with her to ask for these necessary items, she would have returned home without the required prescription. During the visit the physician discussed her condition in technical terms, and when he asked if she took her medicine (which she does not), she replied, "Yes, sir." The examination, conducted with Mrs. Little fully dressed and seated in her wheelchair, consisted simply of his listening to her chest. Similar cursory examinations were observed during visits with Mrs. Washington and Mrs. Finch. Because the hospital is so understaffed, generally no one is available to assist the patient or even be present in the examination room with the physician.

Although Rev. Scott has been receiving regular care at the rheumatology clinic for years, he perceives a decline in the quality of his care and is frustrated by the frequent rotation of physicians. In the passage below he relates a humiliating incident with an unfamiliar physician:

> I've noticed that the rheumatology clinic is not what it's supposed to be. Look like it's hard for them to keep any doctors there. This doctor I had that left and went into private practice asked me if I wanted to go to him, but he was 'way up in northeast Atlanta somewhere. Since then I've gone to a different doctor every time I went down. Last time, I saw a lady doctor that was a foreigner, and I couldn't understand what she was saying. Since I've been having different doctors, I just wrote down the different medicines I was using so I could get a refill on them. I gave them to this little doctor, and she wrote down two or three of them and handed them to me. I said, "I need all of that." [The doctor said:] "I don't have time to

write all of that." Made me wait till she got through waiting on another patient. Some things that happen at County that shouldn't happen. Some don't need their jobs. I guess you can find something like that at most places.

Rev. Scott was able to cope with this situation because he is alert, knowledgeable, and sometimes assertive. He knows what his medications are and can communicate his needs. On the other hand, patients like Eloise Little who encounter similar obstacles very likely return home without their medications.

Another common complaint about County concerns the attitude of the support staff. In the passage below, Sally Finch describes how she felt both ignored and mistreated when she visited the emergency room at County:

> There are some mean old women over there. I was layin' there hurtin'. She come to me, I had slipped on the couch, I was trying to help her, "I think that's the best I can do." She said, "You can do better." When you're hurtin', you don't want no foolishness. They don't pay no attention, do so much talking. Need to get on them about doing their work.

Some of these difficulties encountered by individuals who utilize the public hospital for routine medical care not only undermine the quality of care received but clearly hinder their ability to negotiate the health care system independently. Other studies of minority and inner-city elderly [4-6] have noted similar service delivery elements—long waiting time, confusing atmosphere, not seeing the same doctor twice, insensitivity of doctors and nurses, and lack of effective communication—acting as barriers to satisfactory health care.

In contrast, those participants who go to private physicians believe their health care to be of higher quality and, as a rule, have more satisfying health care experiences. Viola Worth explained how she felt transformed when she switched to private medical care:

> I got tired of the way the doctors [at County] treated me, sent me back like I went. When I changed to Dr. Duncan, I was like a flower bloomed out.

Office visits to private physicians are much less problematic for these disabled elders. This distinction prompted Rev. Scott to search for a private vascular surgeon to care for his chronic leg problems when his condition became so acute he required weekly medical attention:

> Going back there [County] once a week, staying *all* day, I couldn't hardly do that.

Although waits occur in private offices, they are not as long, and usually patients know the staff and can get assistance if they need it.

In addition, the private doctor generally is more experienced, thorough, and familiar with the patient's condition. Geraldine Starr's internist, Dr. Moore, has been treating her for approximately eight years and is well-acquainted with both Mrs. Starr's medical state and her additional long-term care needs. Dr. Moore oversees her care and has referred her to several specialists. During office visits, examinations are thorough, and a nurse is always present to help Mrs. Starr with undressing and dressing and getting on and off the table. If needed, additional tests can be done in the office, or arrangements can be made by the receptionist—a system quite different from the one at County. Mrs. Starr as a rule makes these visits in her wheelchair, unaccompanied, and manages quite well with the assistance provided by staff. She would not, however, be able to negotiate a visit to County, alone, in her present state.

In addition to office visits every three months or so, Mrs. Starr frequently telephones Dr. Moore with questions about her medical condition or her medications, and Dr. Moore regularly writes letters to Medicaid requesting approval for additional drugs and communicates with the RN from the home health service and with Mrs. Starr's regular pharmacist. Such communications are unheard of with County physicians.

Despite the apparent higher quality of care and greater ease of utilization these old people experience with private doctors, some problems, primarily related to personal interactions, still are encountered. Mrs. Starr complains that Dr. Moore, whose typical clientele is white and middle-class, does not give her sufficient time and often attributes this perceived slight to the fact that she is poor and black:

> She does funny to me. I'd like to talk to her woman to woman. There's something about her I like, but she won't let me talk to her like I like. She flies out of the room. She's got so many patients. I want to ask her things. She won't stay in the room long enough. A doctor's not a doctor if he can't talk to you. I've always had doctors I can talk to. She has time to talk to those white people, not colored people I don't think. I want to go to Dr. Jones (her urologist) so bad to talk to him. He's just too nice a person to be a doctor, but he is a doctor.

Rev. Scott also feels slighted by his surgeon:

> He's not the kind of doctor a patient could talk to. I wanted to talk
> to a doctor that would at least listen to what I had to say. My leg is
> not a normal type of leg.

These are complaints common to doctor-patient relationships
with their inherent power differentials, but such perceptions perhaps are heightened when racial differences also are present.
Chubon reported major deficits in understanding between physicians
and mostly elderly rural African Americans, with barriers to communication in both directions [4]. Roberson's study of the meaning of
compliance among a similar population described negative feelings
about doctors in general and about the typical treatment of patients [7].
Obviously the use of private medical care does not eliminate all difficulties, but for these impaired individuals, it does make utilization of care
less burdensome and easier to manage independently and promotes
more productive physician-patient relationships.

## Hospital Visits

Elderly persons are frequent users of acute care services, and this
group is no different. Five of these individuals experienced multiple
acute care episodes during the year-long study period, resulting in
emergency room visits and/or in-patient hospital stays. These episodes
were brought about by either a crisis situation, such as a fall; an
increase in normal symptoms, such as acute pain or elevated blood
pressure; or a secondary development, such as a decubitus ulcer or
infection.

During the year of this study, Lucy Oliver went to the hospital
emergency room six times, for headaches and anxiety over her condition. Eloise Little was an in-patient twice—once in January, for general
weakness, pain, and dehydration, and again in April, for a urinary
tract infection. She visited the emergency room three times for similar
complaints. Geraldine Starr also was hospitalized twice, both times
for surgical procedures—for two days in February to have a
pacemaker implanted and in August for repair and rehabilitation of a
broken hip. The second time she stayed one month in the hospital, a
second month in a specialized rehabilitation hospital, and a third
month in a nursing home. In addition, Mrs. Starr visited the hospital
emergency room on two separate occasions for evaluation, after falls in
her apartment.

Going to a private hospital, although not problem-free, is less stressful than a comparable visit to County. When Mrs. Starr went to the emergency room at a private hospital, her own physician was notified and came to tend to her, and she was back home within a few hours. In contrast, when Mrs. Little was sent to the emergency room at County, she lay there all day and night until she finally was treated by the resident on duty and returned back home at 1 A.M. Similar differences were experienced with in-patient care, such as the presence or absence of appropriate discharge planning.

## FOLLOWING ORDERS

Although physicians believe that compliance is necessary, the extent of non-compliance among patients is high, particularly among patients with chronic conditions requiring long-term treatment regimens [4]. Because elderly persons have more chronic conditions and use more medications, they are among the least compliant patients. Each of these elderly informants is under the care of a physician and, as a rule, abide by prescribed schedules for office and clinic visits. When it comes to following specified health care plans, however, self-care sometimes is defined idiosyncratically. It can be defined even as the decision to do nothing in response to the symptoms of illness.

For these seven elders, like for other patients whose viewpoints have been described in the literature [4, 7, 8,], decisions about compliance are complex. Especially influential for them is the attitudinal dimension, which includes their attitudes toward physicians and toward the role of traditional medical care. While Geraldine Starr is a frequent user of formal health care services and thrives on visits to her doctors, she is influenced as well by her belief in what Wallston and Wallston [9] have described as an external health locus of control. That is, she believes that her personal health is controlled not only by her behavior but also by a higher being, and this belief accounts in part for her failure always to follow instructions. The following passage illustrates her contradictory beliefs:

> I likes 'em [doctors]. I like to go to 'em. I like the experience. I wanted to be a nurse. I've watched a lot of doctor pictures. I've been used to doctors all my life. I reads a lot about the body. I wants to know what's wrong. You're gonna die one day or another. I love for her [Dr. Moore] to talk to me. . . . Some parts of the body supposed to heal itself. The doctor can't heal. I don't know why they mess with people's hearts. That belongs to God. It ain't gonna heal.

Heart, lung, kidneys, bladder, liver—man thinks he can outdo Him but he can't. Just the way it goes. Mess with eyes, it might succeed.

In contrast, Viola Worth regularly follows her physician's instructions, and although, like Mrs. Starr, she too believes a higher being has ultimate power, in her mind the patient shares responsibility and can affect outcomes:

> See, I tells him what I do, you know like sometimes I take Tylenol for pain. The lady [the nurse] asked me about vitamins, and I said I took my own vitamins. My mind led me to take them out there and let them see them. She say these vitamins help strengthen the bone, and I believe it because it looks like to me I can bend sometimes better. But I got in my mind my condition is there, and ain't too much nobody can do about it, except try to work with it. Far as I'm concerned, he's just having me come back and forth to check it. The Master got the doctor there to help us out. You got to have faith in yourself. You can't just depend on the doctors, if you're able, if you're in your right mind.

Eloise Little, on the other hand, characteristically accepts no responsibility and resists all instructions:

> I like 'em [doctors] O.K. Don't like 'em to tell me what to do. I never will get well if I do what they say. Told me to drink that milk, that with the cow on the box. I can't drink that milk.

The attitudes of these seven sick people toward medical authority and toward personal control over their own health interact with other factors—such as lack of money, energy, and social resources—to determine the extent to which their self-care complies with the regimens prescribed for them by health care professionals. These regimens typically include, in addition to hospital and physician visits, prescribed medications, assorted other treatments, and dietary practices.

## Medications

The number of prescribed medications ranges from a low of three for Viola Worth and Joseph Scott to a high of ten for Geraldine Starr. Many of these drugs are prescribed to alleviate certain symptoms, for example, to reduce inflammation and pain or to relieve anxiety and sleeplessness. Others are necessary to prevent more acute conditions or phases of a chronic disease, such as medications for the control of diabetes or hypertension.

Like many older persons, particularly those who live alone, these participants sometimes misuse their drugs, but only Eloise Little chronically misuses all of her prescribed medications. In her case, misuse essentially consists of almost complete lack of use. Of the five to seven medications that are regularly prescribed for her, she rarely takes any of them, and then only when someone puts the medicine and a glass of water in her hand. The drugs, which consist of medications for hypertension, arthritis, gout, heart failure, constipation, and the occasional infection, continue to be prescribed at each clinic visit by physicians ignorant of her non-compliance.

Except for Ms. Worth, each of the other individuals misuses their medications to some extent. As in most studies of non-compliance [10], the most likely categories of medications to be misused are the psychotropic drugs, drugs used to control symptoms, and drugs that produce side effects.

This drug misuse has a number of apparent causes, including mental disorders, lack of knowledge or understanding of a medical condition, dislike for the drug's side effects, failure of the drug to produce the desired result, inability to procure the drug, lack of assistance in administration of the drug, and absence of faith in medical practice.

In the following passage Eloise Little, the most serious non-complier, explains why she does not take her prescribed medications. Although her alcoholism is a major factor in non-compliance, the excuses she offers are based on her lack of trust in the efficacy of a specific medication, as well as her general absence of faith in modern medicine and her need for assistance:

> I hardly ever take it. I forgets. My throat gets all filled up swallowing those big pills, one as big as a biscuit, horse pills. I know I ought to take it. When I think of it, I take all six pills. I don't take it like I should. I know I don't. I takes them every other night—take one night, do for the next. I can't open the bottle. I don't need all those big pills. What am I taking them for? Big old red pills gag me. Water [to take pills] just as warm as pee. I believe in some medicine. That Tylenol don't do any good. I don't want to. They gag me so bad. I'd rather be hurtin'.

Ms. Worth, on the other hand, with her characteristic optimism and a high degree of faith in her prescribed regimen, if not complete knowledge of its function, always takes her medicine as directed:

One for my chest and one for stomach, I think. I don't be knowin'. . . . I *make* myself believe in it. You got to have confidence in what you are doing.

Sally Finch accounts for her underuse of certain drugs by citing the negative side effects she experiences, her fear of addiction, and possible adverse reactions with alcohol. Although she takes her medications for pain and hypertension as directed, she rarely takes a psychoactive drug prescribed to help her sleep and has completely rejected one prescribed for gastrointestinal reflux:

I takes blood pills, water pills, and pain pills. Only thing that keeps me going is those different tablets, but they don't last long. Before you know it, you're hurtin' again. I sticks with it, but I hardly ever takes the one for sleeping. I don't want to get used to 'em [become dependent]. Some nights I get nervous and I take 'em, about five times. I take it likes the directions say, but if I drink me a beer, I don't take none, nothing but the pain pills. I don't think they go together. Sometimes you have to use your own judgement. One medicine they gave me, I like to went crazy—went to the door, change and went to get cold drink, so nervous I don't know what to do, can't sleep, can't lie down. I taken it back to the doctor, "This medicine is running me crazy." He told me just to take a half of one. I came home and put it in the drawer. It's still in there. I'd be crazy if still taking.

Geraldine Starr often gets mixed up taking her many medications, a confusion she attributes to the effect of the drugs themselves, creating a circular problem:

This medicine is doing something to my mind. I had to dial the number two or three times. I sit up here and nod a lot. It sure do work on my mind. My mind just been tore up by these new pills. Half the time I can't remember whether I've taken it or not. My mind's so frizzled. It just slips so quick.

Once she took two diuretics prescribed by different physicians, her regular internist and her urologist. This mishap, however, she blamed on her doctors, which seems an appropriate explanation in this case, as it does for many elderly patients [11]. Mrs. Starr:

It's a pity what these doctors do to old people. I had a bad infected bladder. I know that. Well, hell, I didn't know the other was a water pill. She [her regular doctor] didn't tell me. It said "for swellin'." I called Dr. Jones [the urologist] about water pourin' out of me. Well, *they* was water pills. I was taking two. I didn't think to ask what it was. I hadn't told him. I know it was crazy of me. I generally keeps up with my medicine better. I was hurtin' so bad.

Mrs. Starr also regularly devises her own drug regimen, particularly when troublesome symptoms are not relieved by adhering to her doctor's prescribed plan:

> I takes that Fiber All. That stuff Dr. Moore give don't do any good. She don't want me to take it, but I take it anyway. . . . I told her I ain't taking a half. It's not helping—the little yellow pill, that's supposed to be for my foot pain. It wasn't doing me no good so I been taking a whole one. You know a half a pill don't do nothing for you. I told her, "Dr. Moore, this half a pill ain't helping my feet at all. That's the reason I took a whole one." She forgot I been going to doctors all my life. . . . I had a bad headache yesterday—Lois [her senior companion] told me something that had pressed on my mind. I had taken Anacin all day, but it hadn't helped. Then something said, "Why don't you take two of them Xanax?"—that's what they is, nerve pills—"and lay down to sleep and it'll probably go away." I took it and lay down and read myself to sleep. I woke up this morning and it was gone.

Sometimes these African American elders supplement or replace traditional medicine with folk remedies. When her blood pressure stays up, Ruby Washington drinks garlic water in addition to taking her prescribed medicine, and Mrs. Starr stubbornly sticks to a home remedy for her ears, despite Dr. Moore's instructions to the contrary:

> My ears are dry. Ears are supposed to have wax in 'em. They dry up when you get older. I bought some Sweet Oil to put in 'em. Dr. Moore said not to put it in. I don't see what that would bother, just oil up inside your ear. Old remedies used to be good. People used to use them and get well.

Other research among African Americans has found similar reliance on old-time remedies [7] in preference to more mainstream medical self-care practices.

A regular caregiver can increase drug compliance by helping to obtain medications, to open containers, and to furnish needed reminders and guidance. Mrs. Washington, for one, admits she oftentimes needs her husband to help her remember:

I takes the high blood twice a day, in the morning before I eat and at night. Sometimes I forget, and Jones makes me think about 'em.

Caregivers also can contribute to misuse, as in the case of Lucy Oliver's husband, who has little knowledge of, or faith in, medicine yet often must monitor his wife's medications when she is in a confused state:

That's what pills are for—when they do some good, then leave 'em off. Then take some more of 'em. You know, [if] you keep on taking medicine, nothing do no good.

## Other Treatments

In addition to medications, additional therapeutic procedures or treatments are indicated by the physician or other health care professional for each of these individuals. Such treatments include physical therapy, the use of support stockings, and various remedies to relieve pain and stiffness. Compliance with prescribed regimens is influenced by numerous factors, including attitudes toward health care, medical understanding and knowledge, severity of symptoms, perceived benefits, and access to assistance in carrying out procedures, and is consistent with each person's characteristic drug use behavior. Eloise Little flatly refuses all physical therapy; Viola Worth made every effort to adhere to treatments prescribed after her hip replacement, even after the formal therapy had ceased; and Geraldine Starr complied with the therapeutic regimen at the rehabilitation hospital only as long as it did not require undue effort or discomfort on her part or go against her ingrained beliefs about health care:

My heart ain't taking too much of this pushing. I'm not no young woman, I'm an old woman. My heart's not going to take it. I know my feelings. I know my body better than anybody. They push you too hard. They can't outdo God. They rushing it so. I'm not going to take anybody pushing me too hard. I'm not no slave. You don't push people around 'cause their face is black. They think they can make miracles. They can't make no miracles. It's not going to happen. God don't work that way. Man just has the knowledge, not the power. Why do people want to push you. I wish they'd just leave me alone.

The above passage makes clear the complexity of compliance decisions. Mrs. Starr is genuinely worried about damaging her heart and feels the need to reinforce her status as a sick person. She strongly resists the control of others, particularly of white people over black, and is swayed by her belief that God has supreme control over her health.

While she consistently balks at the use of support hose, at times her failure to follow orders is caused as much by her inability to don them herself as by her obdurate skepticism about their benefits:

> Heck no, I don't wear those stockings! I have a time putting those stockings on. I can't put them things on. Get too old for those things. Dang foolish to try to get an old person to wear something that's against them. If I can get them off, they're coming off. Them things cut your circulation off. Don't know why doctors force those things on you. Why can't they understand? Some do. Dr. Pate at County told me not to wear those wrappers [elastic bandages]. I told Dr. Moore, "I ain't gonna wear something that hurts me. I'm not no young woman. I'm already old." Just can't wear those things. It cuts off my blood. Got the scissors and cut that mess off. I still say it's heart dropsy [the swelling in her legs]. Nothing's going to change my mind.

Sally Finch has similar attitudes about the age-appropriateness of certain health care practices. Despite her submission to regular mammograms at County, she vows she would never agree to surgery:

> Nothing you can do with old age. When you get up in age, all this cuttin' on don't do any good. Nothing to build on. No cuttin' unless a risin' [boil] or something. It might be different if I had somebody to help me.

Her beliefs, too, are influenced by pragmatic assessment of her disability and of her available support.

The need for assistance as a factor in compliance is obviously more significant for those who live alone. Although Mrs. Little resisted physical therapy (which required effort on her part), she welcomes the passive role of being rubbed with liniments, though rarely has anyone around to provide this service. Similarly, Ms. Worth needs help putting her feet in the warm paraffin bath designed to alleviate the pain of arthritis. Rev. Scott was unable to comply with wearing support hose after surgery because he could not put them on by himself. Lack of daily help also dictated the type of bandage he had to wear—the unaboot (a cast-like bandage that stayed in place for two weeks) instead of a gauze dressing that needed daily changing. As with his use of drugs, Rev. Scott's knowledge and understanding of his condition enhances his ability to manage his health care in the most beneficial way. The following passage shows how this understanding influences his self-care activities:

I have said that arthritis is something like an octopus. It kind of squeezes, and you need to do something to break the grip. If you don't continue, it'll come right back and start squeezing again. It's best to be active. If you give up or give in to this arthritis, it's going to get worse. That's the experience I've had. . . . Before I went to Warm Springs, people would try all kinds of rubs on me. I couldn't hardly stand the smell. The doctor told me those rubs couldn't reach my case. The only thing that would help would be moist treatments. I've found since then, if I get out in the sunshine, fresh air, and let that sunshine go into these joints, they'll loosen up.

## Nutrition

For a variety of reasons—including the aging process and chronic disease, a decrease in the quantity of food eaten, insufficiencies of specific nutrients, and various social and economic dynamics—nutritional deficiencies are likely to occur in old age [12, 13]. Among these participants, two, Eloise Little and Sally Finch, are significantly underweight and have been diagnosed as malnourished, though each also points out they were considerably more robust in their younger years. While the other individuals are not underweight, and in fact Mrs. Washington, Mrs. Starr, and Mrs. Oliver are even encouraged by their physicians to lose weight, it is clear that they do not always have a healthy diet.

No one eats the traditional three meals a day. Instead, the usual pattern is breakfast, ranging from only toast and coffee to eggs and bacon, a large meal in the afternoon, and a snack in the evening. The exception to this pattern is Mrs. Little, who rarely has breakfast and whose only dependable meal is her home-delivered meal that comes only on weekdays and, at best, is only partially eaten.

A major factor in nutritional patterns is the older person's ability to shop and prepare meals or the presence of a caregiver to perform these roles. Poverty also limits both the quantity and quality of food that is purchased, especially the number of meals that can be procured from take-out establishments. Rev. Scott likes to order meals from the cafe across the street, but his budget seldom permits him this luxury. In addition, few restaurants locate in, or deliver food to, poor areas. The inferior quality and limited variety of food available at the neighborhood markets further hamper proper nutrition.

Also significant for some is an increasing disinterest in food, either on a regular basis, as expressed by Eloise Little:

> I don't eat much during the day. I don't eat heavy. Bring me enough for two meals, and I have to save some for the next day. I've cut myself down. I be hungry, and I don't be hungry.

. . . or, as Geraldine Starr explains, when the various symptoms of disease are more severe:

> I wasn't hardly able to eat breakfast this morning. At times I don't care whether I eat at all. I'm getting weaker again, and I don't want what I eat.

Dietary restrictions that accompany certain chronic conditions further complicate the nutritional situation. Diabetes dictates not only what Lucy Oliver and Ruby Washington eat, but when and how much. Meals for diabetics should be regular, well-balanced, and coordinated with the taking of medications, and the intake of certain foods is prohibited or restricted. Other common diseases, such as hypertension and related cardiovascular problems, also have nutritional limitations.

All of the above-mentioned factors tend to impede proper nutrition and hinder compliance with dietary restrictions. Mrs. Washington, who has both diabetes and hypertension, tries to follow her diet, but from time to time she succumbs to the temptation of forbidden treats:

> I has a list of foods to eat and a measuring cup. Sometimes I'll eat a little more grits or juice than I'm supposed to. I go down to church, and they have so much good stuff, I have to take a taste, a little potato custard. Sometimes I put a little salt on my food. Don't eat nothing with grease. Most of my chicken is boiled or fried with cooking oil or butter. I don't cook with grease. The doctor at the diabetic clinic wants me to lose twenty-five pounds. I quit eatin' as much—when I eat two biscuits and two pieces of light bread, I cut to one. The doctor don't want me to be fat—messes up my heart.

Sometimes an individual or the caregiver does not fully comprehend dietary matters or is not willing or able to comply, as in the case of Lucy Oliver's husband, who does both the shopping and cooking:

> I saw a sign in the waiting room—"no peppermint candy." I had been giving it to her, a couple of 'em. The diabetic clinic said to give her half apple or half orange. They tell her to use Sweet and Low and diet salt. They try to put [blame] it on what she eat. She might eat too much, but it don't be too salty or too greasy or nothing like that.

Mr. Oliver failed to understand peppermint candy was prohibited, even though he does know his wife is supposed to use artificial sweetener and that the amount and kind of food she eats is critical. Mrs. Oliver, herself, has a better understanding, but sometimes her cognitive impairment interferes with compliance. As the passage below illustrates, she wants to get better and tries to follow orders:

> I been taking those pills and drinking a heap of water. I knowed they told me to drink water, and it would make me better. I hadn't been doing that. I didn't want the water. I believe that's what helped me last week. I started drinking water. I just wanted to do anything I could to help me get well. I'd drink a little and then I'd go back and drink some more.

Those individuals who typically are non-compliant with regard to medications and other therapies exhibit comparable nutrition behavior. Eloise Little freely pours salt over her low-salt home-delivered meal, refuses to wear her dentures, which might alleviate her difficulties with swallowing, and is unusually finicky about her food, often refusing to eat foods prepared for her by her caregivers.

* * * * *

Acute health care services are an important aspect of the long-term care situation we are trying to understand. We have seen in this chapter that the factors determining the medical self-care practices of individuals faced with chronic disease and impairment can be multiple and complex. Though many regimens are prescribed for these seven elders, which ones will be followed and by whom depend heavily on the interaction of a number of elements in their lives. These include their own abilities to manage their health care, their social support, poverty, and race, the health care system available to them, the severity of their disease states and symptoms, motivation, knowledge and understanding of their medical conditions, and their attitudes and beliefs. The choices they make can produce marked improvement in their abilities and outlook, or they can limit or even reverse the benefits available through an imperfect system of care. It is also true, as each person well understands, that certain elements in their lives and conditions cannot be changed appreciably by the self-care behavior they choose.

In Parts II and III, we see the role of the informal and formal support systems in the maintenance of each person's health care regimen. While the role of this support varies, in each case it serves an important function—whether in the form of a simple reminder to take a pill or a long day in the waiting rooms of County Hospital. Next, in Chapter 4, we take a closer look at the day-to-day lives of these seven participants and the impact of their disabilities on their social worlds.

## REFERENCES

1. A. Twaddle and R. Hessler, *A Sociology of Health* (2nd Edition), Macmillan, New York, 1987.
2. K. M. Ness, The Sick Role of the Elderly, in *Psychosocial Nursing Care of the Aged*, I. M. Burnside (ed.), McGraw-Hill, New York, 1980.
3. D. Mechanic, Illness Behavior: An Overview, in *Illness Behavior: A Multidisciplinary Model*, S. McHugh and T. M. Vallis (eds.), Plenum, New York, pp. 101-108, 1986.
4. S. J. Chubon, Personal Descriptions of Compliance by Rural Southern Blacks, *Journal of Compliance in Health Care, 4*:1, pp. 23-38, 1989.
5. M. Cantor and M. Mayer, Factors in Differential Utilization of Services by Urban Elderly, *Journal of Gerontological Social Work, 1*:1, pp. 47-62, 1978.
6. M. K. Petchers and S. Milligan, Access to Health Care in a Black Urban Population, *The Gerontologist, 28*:2, pp. 213-217, 1988.
7. M. H. B. Roberson, The Meaning of Compliance: Patient Perspectives, *Qualitative Health Research, 2*:1, pp. 7-26, 1992.
8. B. W. K. Yee and G. D. Weaver, Ethnic Minorities and Health Promotion: Developing a "Culturally Competent Agenda," *Generations, XVIII*:1, pp. 39-44, 1994.
9. K. Wallston and B. S. Wallston, Health Locus of Control Studies, in *Research with the Locus of Control Concept*, H. Lefcourt (ed.), Vol. 1, Academic Press, New York, pp. 189-243, 1981.
10. F. J. Whittington, Misuse of Legal Drugs and Compliance with Prescription Directions, in *Drugs and the Elderly Adult*, M. D. Glantz, D. M. Petersen, and F. J. Whittington (eds.), U.S. Department of Health and Human Services, Washington, D.C., pp. 63-69, 1983.
11. F. J. Whittington, Drugs, Aging, and Social Policy, in *Drugs and the Elderly: Social and Pharmacological Issues*, D. M. Petersen, F. J. Whittington, and B. P. Payne (eds.), Charles C. Thomas, Springfield, Illinois, 1979.
12. T. Hickey, *Health and Aging*, Brooks-Cole, Monterey, California, 1980.
13. C. A. Rosenbloom and F. J. Whittington, The Effects of Bereavement on Eating Behaviors and Nutrient Intakes in Elderly Widowed Persons, *Journal of Gerontology: Social Sciences, 48*:4, pp. S223-S229, 1993.

# CHAPTER
4

# Social Worlds

*I have myself sort of cut off from the world in a way, not doing what*
*I like to do. I've always been a participator.*

Reverend Joseph Scott

Rev. Scott thrived on the social interactions that his former roles of
Baptist minister and building contractor provided him. He loved
thought-provoking discussions and preaching a stirring sermon. Even
after his accident, when these roles were snatched so abruptly from
him, he still had his wife for ready comfort and conversation and as a
channel to the world outside. Now Rev. Scott is mostly alone, his days
seldom brightened by visitors, telephone calls, or other communal
pleasures.

The frustration expressed by Rev. Scott above is felt by each of the
old people in this book, all of whom have experienced a shrinking of
their social worlds. They are increasingly bound to their homes and,
like many frail elders, often find themselves isolated from family and
friends and from the world outside. The situation is complex and
multidimensional, and a number of factors now present in their lives
unite to create this social deprivation. Functional disabilities restrict
their activities; visible impairments embarrass them; pain and other
vexing symptoms distress them; physical barriers bar access to neighborhoods they are fearful to venture out in; poverty limits opportunities
for transportation and for other kinds of social support; and cultural
attitudes and personalities deter tendencies to reach out. These variables shape the quality of their social lives and the experiences available to each.

The main characters of this book share a bleak prognosis and many
commonalities in the flat routines of their captive lives. They are
unique, however, in the daily rituals and coping strategies they develop

and in the ways they adapt, with varying degrees of success, to their circumscribed worlds.

## HOMEBOUND

The opportunities for these older people to leave their homes have diminished along with their own declining abilities. For Geraldine Starr and Eloise Little, these outings are limited to medical appointments or to hospital stays. Sally Finch sometimes leaves her apartment when the management is spraying for bugs or for a rare trip to the trash drop down the hall or to her mail box downstairs. Rev. Scott and Ruby Washington at times attend church. Lucy Oliver attends an adult day rehabilitation center three days each week. Only Viola Worth has regular outings to go shopping or to the beauty shop.

As Schulz and Williamson point out, the magnitude of the negative effects of the stress associated with a disabling condition is greater to the extent that it restricts normal activities [1]. The distress caused by this confinement is especially severe for Mrs. Starr, who despairs over her inability to come and go as she pleases:

> What got me cramped down is not being able to get out. I wishes I could get out of here. Don't get to go but one place—Dr. Moore's. I actually don't want to live if I can't go out by myself and come back by myself. I didn't mind being by myself till I got where I couldn't get out.

In addition to lacking the freedom to come and go and to take care of needs outside the home, these elders miss experiencing the world outside. Before his problems with leg ulcers developed, Rev. Scott occasionally could go for brief outings in his car, to McDonald's, to watch football practice at a nearby high school, or just to sight-see. He now complains of "housitis" and longs "to be free" of his house. Mrs. Starr explains how she feels insulated from life in her highrise:

> Can't see nothing from in here. I'd like to be where I could see Marta [the metropolitan rapid transit train] go by, see some people. All I can see is trees.

For those who lament their insular lives, an opportunity simply to leave home is welcome. On a rare shopping trip, Mrs. Starr proclaimed:

> Just fly away! I'm going to sit back and enjoy it. How wonderful!

Ms. Worth expresses a common view:

I just want to go! [You] can't learn something staying at home all
the time.

In a qualitative study of very old people (85 years old) in Sweden,
Carlsson-Agren and associates found that just getting out of the house
was for them a major component of experiencing a good day [2].
Moreover, people who are shut-in often experience a real sensory
deprivation. Lustbader has likened a social outing for a homebound
person to a "sensual circus," an apt metaphor for these old people [3].

For some, it is the reduced social interactions that often accompany
being housebound that are especially bothersome. Mrs. Little, who is
often alone, misses most being around other people:

I sure wish I could go. When I lived in the project, I could jump out
and go to somebody's house, talk to them. I'd feel like a new person.

And when Mrs. Washington can get to her church the experience also
is therapeutic:

I always joined a church close to me. I feel good myself. I pat my
hands.

Getting out for these old people is difficult for several reasons. The
level of impairment obviously limits not only the ability to leave the
house alone but also the ease with which others are able to take them.
The availability of social support is also a factor, as is their poverty and
that of some caregivers. Viola Worth gets out more because, with the
aid of her walker, she can go out of her house and down to the street
and get in and out of cars unassisted. She also has a walker that folds
(a type not paid for by Medicaid) and a support system that includes
helpers willing to take her places. In a typical month Ms. Worth might
make her regular visit to the post office to get her check, go on one or
two shopping trips, visit the beauty parlor, attend church, and go to the
doctor.

For the others, who must have wheelchairs to go out, leaving home
obviously is more problematic, particularly when their homes have
environmental barriers. Rev. Scott can go no further than his side
porch in his wheelchair and has only one informal helper who is able to
take him out regularly. These trips are restricted to frequent medical
appointments and an occasional Sunday at church.

Ruby Washington's social outings are limited to places she can be
pushed in her wheelchair, since she has no regular caregivers who own
a car. She goes to church when her health and the weather permit,
about twice a month.

Even for Geraldine Starr and Sally Finch, who live in apartments specifically built for persons who are elderly and handicapped, environmental barriers limit access to the outer world. Neither of these women is able to negotiate the heavy, non-automatic doors that are standard in low-income highrises, and weakness limits the distances they are able to propel themselves in their wheelchairs.

Even when the means to leave home is available, troublesome symptoms can discourage the inclination to venture out. Pain or urinary problems are a common deterrent. Ms. Worth, who loves to be around people and used to participate regularly in group activities, hesitates to go places where she might not be able to lie down or find a bathroom when the need arises. Difficulties in getting ready to go out, such as getting dressed or bathing, create additional barriers, especially if no one is available to help and if mental or emotional difficulties, such as anxiety, are also present.

Other studies have found that fear of crime is a factor that commonly limits the activities of frail elders who live in unsafe neighborhoods, particularly in urban environments [4, 5]. Such fears certainly contribute to the seclusion of these participants. Although Mrs. Finch lives in a highrise with a security guard, she is fearful even of going out into the hall or answering her door after dark:

> I'm scared to go out by myself. When night comes, I don't even go out in the hall, unless the fire alarm goes off. Every now and then I go to the dumpster to empty my garbage, when I forget to ask the nurse [aide] [to empty it for me], but I don't go out by myself. There too many strange people. It's scary.

Mr. Oliver explains how frequent violence in their public housing project keeps Mrs. Oliver inside:

> I can't even leave my wife on the porch. Can't ever tell when they're going to start shooting.

Ruby Washington is afraid to leave her home for fear of losing her few possessions. She quit attending a day program because she was burglarized on several occasions, and more recently her Social Security check was stolen while she went to the hospital for a few nights.

More subjective factors, such as embarrassment about one's condition, also play a key role in decisions of these elders to stay home. Rev. Scott, who as a Baptist minister was always active in his church, chose to remain sequestered when his leg problems kept him from wearing a shoe:

> I'd rather not go out like that. I wasn't sick as such. I didn't feel like showing my toes. I wouldn't have felt right.

Lucy Oliver also shuns church because it is customary for the wife of a minister (Mr. Oliver is a lay-minister in the Baptist church) to speak during the service, and people sometimes laughed at her speech handicap:

> They make fun of you or talk about you. They ashamed of me I guess.

Matthews [6] found similar inclinations to avoid threatening situations among older widows with diminished capacities, and Schulz and Williamson [1] noted the negative impact of the visibility of disability on social interactions.

Viola Worth, however, refuses to let her handicap diminish her self-esteem. The outward signs of her impairment are not as dramatic, and perhaps because she has been impaired all her life, she is less bothered by the impact of her condition on others. Rubinstein suggests that continuity of personal identity is key—persons who have experienced poor health or physical handicap from an early age and have adapted successfully to these identities find later health changes to be less threatening to self-image [4]. Schulz and Williamson also point out that the impact of illness varies as a function of the elapsed time since onset [1].

For two of these participants, Geraldine Starr and Sally Finch, the threat of uncomfortable or upsetting encounters is compounded by long-held cultural values and personalities that discourage social interaction. While their confinement is stressful and often lonely, they typically choose solitude over participation in group activities or socializing with other residents in their highrises. Mrs. Starr explains her reclusive behavior:

> I don't want to be bothered with these folks. They ask you such stupid damn questions. I went out the other day and they didn't speak right away. Then they spoke. "What you speaking now for?" They're sometimey. One time eat you up, next time don't speak. I'll stay in here and keep my bills together. Not that I think I'm better. I get tired of gossiping. That's children's stuff, tease one another. Next thing you know they're cussing, next thing about to fight. No need of me mongling with them. I can listen to my radio, read a magazine, read my Bible. I just wasn't raised up that way. We stayed at home.

Mrs. Finch, often nervous and anxious, offers similar justifications for staying in:

I get along better not going in and out of apartments. I enjoy being alone. My nerves are bad. Best to stay in your own apartment. I've been here five years and haven't been in but one apartment. I know a few people and a few people know me, but they never tell me to come and see them, so I don't go. 'Course I never did believe in people running in and out, never did. Some speak and some don't. Some of them can't help it, but some of them is so mean. When you get old you're supposed to be sweeter, you know, to each other. That's how come I stay up here. They wants to know your business. Your back is turned, they talk about you. I stay up here and mind my own business. There's some mean old people. I'm already down and my feelings are easy to hurt 'cause I'm down already. I was down in the wash room one day, to wash some pajamas out. Two ladies were there. One started pickin' at me, telling me where to sit. Made me mad. I rolled out in the hall and sat there. I'm not supposed to get mad. My blood pressure just shot up, my head started pounding. I didn't say nothing to her. Sometimes people think they more than you. She looked like a hag if I do say so myself. If they ain't bothering you, don't bother them. That's why I stay to myself. I don't like too much bossing after I done got older. Different ones want to be bosses. Best to stay out of there. Doctor told me that when I had my nervous breakdown, to stay out of crowds as much as possible. Hard to get along with a crowd of people, but I can get along with the devil. I was brought up to be quiet and stay at home.

For Mrs. Finch, being around people, especially in groups, intensifies her symptoms. She tries to reduce her anxiety and protect an already damaged self-image by avoiding conflictual encounters. Continuity of personal identity is relevant for Mrs. Starr and Mrs. Finch. Both self-proclaimed loners, they display behavior patterns reinforced by life-long habits and beliefs. We found their reclusive behavior akin to that of the marginal residents described in other studies of urban highrises [5-7].

In addition to avoiding contact, these two women try to increase their social distance from other residents by establishing a negative identification with them. A similar strategy was described by Myerhoff in her study of old Jewish people [8]. Each proclaims who she is (a loner) by asserting who she is not (child, gossiper, hag, mean old person), and this identification helps justify the decision to remain isolated. According to Myerhoff, by emphasizing their distances and differences, the elderly Jews in her study were "saved from seeing themselves reflected in their peers, most of whom they regarded as weak, pathetic, and lonely" [8, p. 184]. They thus set themselves above and apart from those they thought to be inferior. This notion of "relative deprivation" was applied to nursing home residents by Savishinsky when he described residents without cognitive impairment who distanced themselves from residents with dementia [9].

Similar strategies are described by Karen Rook, in her discussion of strains in older adults' friendships [10]. Rook suggested that people with low self-esteem sometimes adopt dysfunctional interpersonal strategies in order to minimize the risk of negative feedback. Mrs. Starr and Mrs. Finch regularly employ two of the strategies she cites—rebellion, which serves to invalidate others as a source of negative feedback, and social withdrawal, a way of reducing the threat of rejection by eliminating contact completely.

Rose Shield observed nursing home residents who used conflict with each other to guard against closeness [11]. She explained their motives for remaining aloof from one another in terms of the desire to preserve autonomy. A key factor in the choice of this strategy was their inability to reciprocate in social relationships. We will see in Chapters 6 and 7 that spurning social ties sometimes is a strategy used by these two women to maintain their independence.

These alternative ways of interpreting behaviors help explain why anti-social affirmations do not always ring true. For when Geraldine Starr makes a trip to her doctor, she turns on the charm for the nurses and for the clerks in the drugstore where she waits for her ride, trying to establish relationships. Even Mrs. Finch has expressed pleasure about a visit to the community room while her apartment was being sprayed:

> I really enjoyed it. [I] didn't want to come home. Talk about old times.

Their claims of preferred solitude may serve as rationalizations for what often cannot be. Perhaps, as Rubinstein suggested, continuity of personal identity can also be re-interpreted to fit present circumstances [4]. Sally Finch rationalizes her behavior by explaining that she was "brought up to stay at home" because she now feels she has no other alternative.

Compounding these barriers related to physical frailty, poverty, personality, and reclusive attitudes, is the reluctance of the dependent person to "bother" would-be helpers—to be a burden. Such feelings contribute to Mrs. Oliver's decision to stay home from church. When her husband still had his car, he could take her to her own church, where she felt more comfortable and was not expected to speak publicly, but she now has to depend on others for a ride:

People don't want to bother with you when you get old. I'm used to going. When we had a car, my husband could take me to church. I used to go all the time. Now I can't go.

Mrs. Finch's tendency to remain isolated is encouraged by a similar attitude. Staying home now has become a habit:

I hardly ever go downstairs. I feel like I'm a burden so I don't worry them unless I have to. I feel like I'm in the way. I don't want nobody to be bothered with me, pushing [in her wheelchair]. I'd just as soon stay here. I done stayed home so long I don't care whether I go or not.

These attitudes toward dependence and being helped will be further analyzed in Part II when we examine the impact of social support systems on the lives of these seven elders.

## FRIENDS AND VISITORS

Social research upholds the importance of interaction with friends as a source of social integration into the community and broader society [12]. For these participants, particularly those who live alone, the isolation caused by not getting out is coupled with a corresponding reduction in friends and visitors. Only Mrs. Washington and Ms. Worth identify close friends. The others rarely even have outside visitors.

The association between declining health and a reduction in friendships is well-documented in the literature [10, 13-15]. It is an association acknowledged by certain of these elders, who believe their impairments have precipitated the loss of friends. Rev. Scott attributes the desertion of his friends, whose visits and conversation he sorely misses, to his accident and subsequent dependency:

A lot of people I considered my friends changed on me after that happened. I know two people I thought were my friends didn't want no part of me after the accident. For instance, I think of some of the ministers I was in seminary with. I thought they were my friends. After I got hurt, none of them came to see me. When a person becomes disabled, people don't visit them often, even people you know well. Weeks at a time, nobody stops by or even calls. Well so many people who could just pass by, a little something they could do to help. Don't know whether they thought I wanted something from them. I just wanted to talk.

Mrs. Finch, who claims to have no friends, shares this viewpoint:

> When you're on your feet, you have some friends. So-called friends throw you down [when you are disabled].

The loss of friends that frail elders often experience is precipitated in part by their failed capacities to nurture friendships. Numerous studies cite the importance of reciprocity in the maintenance of friendships and also in whether friendships are beneficial to well-being [10, 12, 15, 16]. Although research validates the contribution of friendship to morale and well-being in old age [12], inequitable relationships—where participants are both overbenefited and under-benefited—have been linked to feelings of anger, discontent, and loneliness [17, 18]. Illness and disability frequently create demands for a level of support that exceeds the resources of friends, while at the same time reducing the opportunities of dependent persons to reciprocate [10, 15]. As we see in subsequent chapters, the ability of these seven older people to reciprocate in their relationships is not only a crucial determinant of their affective bonds with their informal caregivers but is often a determining factor in whether they are able to garner the more instrumental help they each need. They often are unwilling to reach out to those who might help because they have little to offer in return. As Roberto noted, we see that an individual's personality can influence the degree of significance attached to equity in relationships [17].

An additional barrier to having close friends and regular visitors is the corresponding impairment of members of their social networks, many of whom also are elderly. Sally Finch's former friends from her old neighborhood no longer are able to get around, and her sister also is homebound. Rev. Scott's only sister in town is in a nursing home. Johnson and Troll identified increased age of friends as one of four factors constraining friendships in a sample of elders eighty-five years and older [15]. On the other hand, when friends have similar frailties, they too lack opportunities to reciprocate, and relationships are thus more balanced. As Dowd suggested, exchange relations tend to form among partners of similar power [18]. In such cases, ties sometimes remain quite close, being nurtured principally through frequent telephone visits. This is one way Ms. Worth and Mrs. Washington maintain closeness with their friends.

Certain of these old people, however, have greater resources for social interactions and relationships. The businesses of Viola Worth and Joseph Scott, for example, have the latent function of bringing people into their homes. Neighbors stop by most days to buy drinks from Ms. Worth, and on game nights she holds court on her porch while "watching" her cars and talking to passersby. She now counts some of her "parkers" among her friends. During tax season Rev. Scott's customers provide welcome company, if not friendship:

> I always get a bit of enjoyment when people come in during the tax season. Some of 'em come in and want to talk and haven't seen 'em in about a year. Someone came in today had some papers he wanted me to fill out. One old man in his nineties came trying to tease me. I tease him sometime too, ask him if he's still single. I kind of got his dander up about getting married. His wife died a few years back.

Those who are church members—Rev. Scott, Mrs. Oliver, Ms. Worth, and Mrs. Washington—also have additional opportunities for social contacts. Although visitors still are not frequent, they have a wider circle of acquaintances, and church members occasionally stop by on the weekends.

As with leaving home, the desire to have people visit is influenced by the symptoms of disease. Those people who are depressed, in pain, or having incontinence problems often prefer to be alone. Such symptoms reinforce the antisocial tendencies of Geraldine Starr and Sally Finch, who frequently grumble about the few visitors they do have. Mrs. Finch complains that her niece's children always bother her belongings and that she has to clean up after they leave. Mrs. Starr similarly fusses that people "get on her nerves" or cause her to be confused about her medicine:

> That's the reason I'd rather be by myself. I can concentrate better, I can think better. I can just about tend to all my business myself. What I can't, I ask the Lord to help.

Although numerous studies depict age-segregated highrises as community-like places where friendships are common and frequent visiting takes place [19-22], each of these studies also described aloof tenants who, like Mrs. Finch and Mrs. Starr, eschew close ties. A convivial person akin to Viola Worth, however, is unequivocal about her welcome of social interactions:

> I like people, period!

And Rev. Scott makes explicit his longings for more opportunities for conversation:

I think about that sometime when I'm here by myself alot and don't have anyone to talk to, that I might forget how to communicate. I always enjoy talking to people.

Johnson and Troll point out that personality traits, such as gregariousness, remain stable throughout life and encourage patterns of sociability whenever possible [15]. Affective ties clearly are an important source of meaning for Ms. Worth. Like one of the old people that Kaufman so vividly described in her study of the sources of meaning in old age [23], Ms. Worth frequently explains herself in terms of her talent for getting along with other people and making friends. We see in later chapters that this skill serves her well when trying to increase her networks of support.

## DAILY LIFE

So how do these seven frail elders experience an ordinary day? How do they cope with decreasing social interactions and being homebound, and how do they pass the time?

In the following passage, Ms. Worth, the most physically able one of this group, portrays the routine quality of her everyday life:

I just get up and do whatsonever [sic] I feel like doing. I don't have no special time to get up. If I'm not resting good, I'm subject to get up at six o'clock, seven o'clock, anytime. Usually, to really call myself getting up and getting started, giving God thanks like I do before I get up, all depend on how I feel and what I want to do, I hit the floor around seven, that is if I ain't going nowhere. If I'm looking for [expecting] my aide and if I got something to do, I get up and I get started. A lot of time when she get here I done washed. My regular time for getting up, my days when nobody come, I get up and I stir around. So I don't have nothing to do. I sit around, listen to T.V. I sit in the kitchen. If got some cooking to do, I do that. I don't have nothing special, just no special nothing, just my regular routine, whatever I feel up to doing, whether it's cooking, washing, trying to clean. If the weather's beautiful enough, I may end up outdoors, if it ain't nothing but go out there and come down the side of the house, 'cause I stay in so much I feel like I need air. I just be stirring and be thankful I'm able to stir.

A typical day for Ms. Worth is "just no special nothing," an apt description of the days at home for each of these participants with similar rhythm and content in their lives. Still, she, and they, have their daily routines.

As revealed in previous chapters, activities of daily living can occupy a good portion of a day, and each person has a preferred schedule. Allocation of time to these routine tasks, and to other daily pastimes, depends on each individual's personal resources and preferences, as well as on the needs that the activities fulfill. While performing activities of daily living has the obvious function of meeting basic needs, these activities also have latent benefits. For Mrs. Finch, performing these chores helps to pass time and provides relief from loneliness and anxiety:

> Most of the time I just straighten up to keep my mind together. Don't have much company. Sometimes I get so lonely, I start to cleaning. It be's so quiet.

Intellectual capacities afford other participants additional means of passing time. Rev. Scott's accounting skills allow him to still work despite his limited mobility. When his endurance is limited, as it often is, more essential tasks take precedence:

> I work according to how I feel. If I'm not feeling well I put everything aside. Still have to have time to warm up a little food, fix me something to eat. If I work two or three days pretty hard straight for several hours, I feel sort of like resting a day or two. I haven't gotten into it like I did in previous years.

Rev. Scott also spends time reading, substituting literary characters for the visitors he misses:

> I try to stay busy, find me something to read sometime and talk with the people in the book, let them talk to you. I get tired of watching TV and playing radio.

Mrs. Starr too enjoys reading—the daily paper ("like a book, section by section") her Bible every night, assorted religious and health pamphlets, and, when she has a chance to buy them, *True Confessions, The National Enquirer,* and detective magazines. Mrs. Starr said she would be "walking around crying" if kept from this cherished diversion. The other five participants never spend time reading because they either lack the intellectual skills, or they have visual or mental impairments that intervene.

For some, talking on the telephone helps pass time and is a vital means of preserving social ties. In some cases the telephone may be the only avenue of contact with family and friends, or with anyone, for several days. Mrs. Washington often fills her evening hours talking to members of her social network:

> I don't stay up much at night. Sometimes I go to bed at six o'clock and take a nap, and then I wake up about ten o'clock and I stay woke, talk to my friends on the telephone. They stays up till the news comes on and afterwards. My brother and his wife stays up till nearly eleven-thirty, and my cousin, she stays up. I calls them and they calls me. We have a time talking when we all get woke.

Barriers relating to frailty or economic circumstances may impede even this pastime and mode of social interaction. Mrs. Oliver and Mrs. Little have difficulties dialing and remembering numbers, and Mrs. Oliver's speech impediment is a further hindrance. Mrs. Little often gets relief from just talking to herself:

> That's my company. I talk to Eloise [herself] all the time. Ain't got anybody to talk to. Better off. I like that. I really do. I love it. Get it off your mind.

Rev. Scott explains how his limited income restricts phone calls to his sisters who live out of town:

> About my sister in LaGrange, she gets wound up talking. Last time we talked it was $10. She's a talker once she gets started. They want me to do all the calling. So I don't call often. Her health isn't too good right now. She used to come up here but she doesn't do that anymore. She had a fall this summer.

And Mrs. Starr's difficulties with mobility cause her sometimes to discourage would-be callers:

> I get so nervous I be shakin' all over. I can't get to it. It gets on your nerves so bad. I get hemmed up in there [the bathroom]. I tell 'em, just shut up and don't call me no more.

Television viewing plays an important role in some of these lives. It is a source of information about the world outside, a distraction from worry, noise to fill the silence, as well as a way to occupy time. Individual attitudes, however, govern its legitimacy as a diversion. For Mrs. Starr:

> I play that thing night and day. That's my company. I wake up
> listening to it. I mostly watch cartoons. Get more thrill out of it
> than that mess [soap operas]. Some of it reminds me of my own life.

Ms. Worth, on the other hand, disapproves of continuous TV watching,
especially if she has work to do. She often keeps it turned on, but she is
careful to distance herself from others who devote too much time to this
pastime:

> I look at them [programs] in the mornings mostly than I do any-
> thing else, but if I have something to do, the TV just be on and I'm
> going on about my business. I don't see how these women, some of
> 'em with these soap operas and all. No wonder they having these
> babies, lay there cooking these quick meals, throw something
> together. I can't do my work like that. When I was working, I liked
> to go on and get my work done.

Mrs. Finch expressed a similar view:

> Lots of time I have it on but don't pay no attention, be doing
> something else. Some sit *all* day and watch. I couldn't.

Rev. Scott watches TV only at night after he gets in bed. For him
television is no substitute for the family gatherings filled with conversation he so wistfully remembers:

> I have said that these TV's and stereos are designed to distract
> rather than unify life. There are times when you need a unifying
> force in your life, and you can't get that from the TV. When you
> didn't have those things, people would gather as a family at night
> where they'd have a chance to talk to each other. Now they don't
> have time to talk to each other, just looking at TV all the time.

Except for Mrs. Oliver and Mrs. Little, who doze off regularly—
aided by medication and alcohol—sleeping is not a routine part of daily
life for these old people. Ms. Worth does not have "time to nap," and
even Mrs. Washington, who spends most of her days in bed, rarely
does:

> Sometimes I take a nap, if I don't have nothing to do. Time sure do
> get away.

Tobacco and alcohol provide, for some, additional coping
mechanisms to deal with social isolation and fill time. Mrs. Finch is

the only smoker, and while she claims to prefer solitude, she calls cigarettes her "company keepers":

> Can't do without, just get in the habit. I have tried to give it up. Be so lonesome. If I didn't have a cigarette, I don't know what I'd do.

The other women all use snuff, more heavily when they are alone, and Mrs. Little, and occasionally Mrs. Finch, also drink beer.

All in all, despite the restricted social environments and the limited alternatives for passing time, time does not drag by for these seven elders. Rather, as Mrs. Washington puts it, "it sure do get away." One day is usually just like the one before, but somehow the hours of each day are filled. For Rev. Scott, who has several viable alternatives:

> I usually find something to do all summer long. If I don't get interested in reading or studying, I might draw some blueprints for somebody.

And for Mrs. Little, who has few choices:

> I can find something to do all the time, if it ain't nothing but straightening them baskets out.

In its sameness, each life has a degree of structure and each person a preferred routine. Other research has suggested that such *ritualization* of daily life helps sustain self-control and promote psychological and physical well-being [2]. These authors noted that clients' personal timetables must be considered carefully when planning care interventions in order to preserve the highest level of autonomy. We see in later chapters that caregiving schedules are not always sensitive to the daily routines of these seven elders, who value highly their independence.

* * * * *

We have seen that daily life for these seven African American elders often is an insular experience. Numerous impediments—physical impairment, environmental barriers, embarrassment, lack of social support, fear of crime, and poverty—keep them increasingly housebound and interfere with their previous avenues of social integration. For some people these obstacles fuse with attitudes and beliefs—

some life-long and some born out of the deterioration of their bodies—to contribute to further isolation. Although not every participant is alone or lonely, everyone's social world is diminished.

In many instances, what makes the social isolation of these participants most distressing is its combination with frailty and dependence. It is being alone *and* not being able to take care of needs independently or carry out accustomed activities that causes the greatest despair. With persistent regularity, each day delivers anew unabated challenges and wearisome routines. While they aspire to self-reliance in their daily lives, the reality often is the need for assistance.

In the remainder of the book, we examine the role of social support in the lives of these seven African American elders. First, we explore the care supplied by family and friends—the informal caregiving system. Then we turn to the formal care system. With each system, we pay attention to how well it meets the needs of these elderly participants and to the factors that modify and influence the effectiveness of each. Particular consideration will be given to the role of the dependent person in the management and control of care. The problems of dependency and of being helped are recurring themes.

## REFERENCES

1. R. Schulz and G. M. Williamson, Psychosocial and Behavioral Dimensions of Physical Frailty, *Journal of Gerontology, 48*:Supplement, pp. 39-43, 1993.
2. M. Carlsson-Agren, S. Berg, and C. G. Wenestam, Daily Life of the Oldest Old, *Journal of Sociology & Social Welfare, 19*:2, pp. 109-124, 1992.
3. W. Lustbader, *Counting on Kindness: The Dilemmas of Dependency*, The Free Press, New York, 1991.
4. R. L. Rubinstein, J. C. Kilbride, and S. Nagy, *Elders Living Alone*, Aldine de Gruyter, New York, 1992.
5. J. Smithers, *Determined Survivors: Community Life Among the Urban Elderly*, Rutgers University Press, New Brunswick, New Jersey, 1985.
6. S. Matthews, *The Social World of Old Women: Management of Self-Identity,* Sage Publications, Inc., Beverly Hills, California, 1979.
7. J. F. Gubrium, *The Mosaic of Care*, Springer, New York, 1991.
8. C. Cohen and J. Sokolovsky, Social Engagement versus Isolation: The Case of the Aged in SRO Hotels, *The Gerontologist, 20*, pp. 36-40, 1980.
9. B. Myerhoff, *Number Our Days*, Simon & Schuster, New York, 1978.
10. J. Savishinsky, *The Ends of Time: Life and Work in a Nursing Home*, Bergin and Garvey, New York, 1991.
11. K. S. Rook, Strains in Older Adults' Friendships, in *Older Adult Friendships*, R. G. Adams and R. Blieszner (eds.), Sage Publications, Inc., Newbury Park, California, 1989.

12. R. Shield, *Uneasy Endings: Daily Life in an American Nursing Home*, Cornell University Press, Ithaca, New York, 1988.
13. S. E. Crohan and T. C. Antonucci, Friends as a Source of Social Support in Old Age, in *Older Adult Friendships*, R. G. Adams and R. Blieszner (eds.), Sage Publications, Inc., Newbury Park, California, 1989.
14. G. A. Allan and R. G. Adams, Aging and the Structure of Friendship, in *Older Adult Friendships*, R. G. Adams and R. Blieszner (eds.), Sage Publications, Inc., Newbury Park, California, 1989.
15. P. O'Conner, Same-Gender and Cross-Gender Friendships among the Frail Elderly, *The Gerontologist, 33*, pp. 24-30, 1993.
16. C. L. Johnson and L. E. Troll, Constraints and Facilitators to Friendships in Late Late Life, *The Gerontologist, 34*:1, pp. 79-87, 1994.
17. K. Roberto and J. Scott, Equity Considerations in Friendships of Older Adults, *Journal of Gerontology, 41*, pp. 241-247, 1986.
18. K. A. Roberto, Equity in Friendships, in *Older Adult Friendships*, R. G. Adams and R. Blieszner (eds.), Sage Publications, Inc., Newbury Park, California, 1986.
19. J. D. Dowd, *Stratification Among the Aged*, Wadsworth, Belmont, California, 1980.
20. A. Hochschild, *The Unexpected Community*, Prentice Hall, Englewood Cliffs, New Jersey, 1973.
21. E. Wellin and E. Boyer, Adjustments of Black and White Elderly to the Same Adaptive Niche, *Anthropological Quarterly, 52*, pp. 39-46, 1979.
22. K. Jonas, Factors in the Development of Community among Elderly Persons in Age-Segregated Housing: Relationships between Involvement in Friendship Roles with the Community and External Social Roles, *Anthropological Quarterly, 52*, pp. 29-38, 1979.
23. J. K. Ross, *Old People, New Lives: Community Creation in a Retirement Residence*, University of Chicago Press, Chicago, 1977.
24. S. Kaufman, *The Ageless Self: Sources of Meaning in Late Life*, The University of Wisconsin Press, Madison, Wisconsin, 1986.

# Part II
# The Informal Care Experience

# CHAPTER
5

# Family and Friends

*I don't have anybody to do anything for me. When my sister was living she used to send somebody whenever I needed help. I don't have any kinfolks in Atlanta. Heap of 'em I've done for all my life, have called me for help. God knows I've done all I could. I've made ceramic dogs and cats at the center and given to them. I called them and they didn't come. God will take care of me. I've been here without a mouth[ful] to eat or a drop of water.*

Eloise Little

Eloise Little assesses her situation accurately. Even though she sometimes is too weak even to sit up in bed, she has no family or friends she can really count on to help her everyday. She has no one to fix regular meals, shop, bathe her, do laundry, clean house, change her bed, cash her checks, assist with medications, or provide transportation and accompany her to County Hospital for her regular clinic appointments. Older persons like her—unmarried and childless—are the most likely to share her predicament.

Estimates indicate that from 60 to 85 percent of all impaired older persons are helped by informal care in some significant way. It is this support from family and friends, not professionals, that provide the bulk of care to impaired elderly persons and often even prevents institutionalization [1]. Despite this resounding affirmation of the role of family and friends, some older persons like Mrs. Little remain isolated, without even minimal informal support [2-5].

Of the seven elders in this book, only Mrs. Washington and Mrs. Oliver are married, Mrs. Oliver to her husband of more than fifty years and Mrs. Washington to her common-law husband, Mr. Jones. Except for Ms. Worth who never married, the others have been without their spouses for at least five years, Mrs. Little and Mrs. Finch for over thirty.

In addition to their spouses, Mrs. Oliver and Mrs. Washington have at least one child available to give regular care. Mrs. Oliver has seven children living in town, and Mrs. Washington's son, Robert, lives in one side of her house. The others are not so fortunate. Mrs. Starr has lost contact with her two sons, and Ms. Worth is estranged from her son, only hearing from him on holidays and special occasions. Mrs. Little's only son died many years ago, and Mrs. Finch and Rev. Scott never had children.

Five of this group of seven old people can be considered among that most vulnerable sector of the elderly population, those who are childless—or effectively so—and unmarried. These same five have few other relatives available. Four of them also live alone. These social characteristics assure their membership in the group of frail elderly persons most at risk of institutionalization [6-8].

The abundance of literature that speaks to the critical role of informal support in the care of frail old people offers little evidence of shared responsibility within the kinship network. Numerous writers have suggested instead that a "principle of substitution" operates whereby old people turn first to spouses, then to children and other relatives, and finally to friends and neighbors [2, 7, 9, 10]. Research has confirmed the operation of this principle also among African American families [11, 12].

Among elderly persons who are married, the spouse is the primary care provider. The marital dyad relies almost totally on each other for care, turning to other family members only when no spouse is present or when the needs for assistance exceed the capability of the caregiving spouse [5, 7, 13-16]. Although married women assume the caregiving role more frequently than men [17], men may take on this traditionally female role [18].

The signiflcant contribution (both instrumental and emotional) by children to their elderly parents also is widely reported in the literature (2, 16, 19-23]. Care from children ranges from minimal help with tasks of daily living to comprehensive care of bedfast parents. Among African American families the critical role of support from children is well documented [2, 24-29].

As the literature suggests, the two women in this study with spouses and children available, Mrs. Washington and Mrs. Oliver, fare much better than Mrs. Little. Though both are significantly disabled, most of their basic needs are met by their spouses. These same two women also have children who play a less supportive role, but who still feel an obligation to help. Of the seven participants, they alone have informal caregivers who regularly perform personal care tasks, a finding consistent with other evidence that only spouses and female members of the same household or living close by are likely to perform these services [30].

Siblings, other relatives, and friends are most likely to provide only socio-emotional support [26, 31]. Although reports of the day-to-day care of impaired elders by these groups of helpers exist [5, 14, 32-35], especially in age-segregated settings [34, 35], generally they cannot be counted on for such committed care [36].

Previous research anticipates that the five participants who have no spouses or children available also have no primary caregivers. One person, Mrs. Starr, has no regular informal support at all. When siblings or more distant kin do provide care, they assume no major instrumental roles. Mrs. Finch's sister-in-law shops for groceries monthly, and Rev. Scott's brother and niece only occasionally help out. Siblings for the most part offer only socio-emotional support such as daily phone calls between Mrs. Finch and her sister. Yet, for those with surviving siblings, the sibling relationship is the strongest bond. These findings support other studies of childless elderly persons [14] and of family support among community-dwelling African Americans [26, 37].

The care received by these African American elders from friends and neighbors reflects the normative, more limited role generally found in other research. A few people have regular support from these kinds of helpers, but only Rev. Scott's friend, Deacon Pate assumes a significant caregiving role. Even the highrise settings, which often have been found to promote interdependent relationships, offer just one lone example of regular helping.

Those people with church ties, however, do show increased opportunities for both instrumental and emotional support, exemplifying supportive situations commonly reported among black congregations [12, 24, 26, 38, 39].

Ms. Worth is the only person who has regular support from fictive kin—non-family members who take the place of her absent or unsatisfactory blood relations [40]. The use of fictive kin as informal helpers has been described in other studies of both African American and white families [23, 26, 36, 41-43].

While some of the differences in the informal networks of support can be accounted for by the availability of close kin, such as spouses and children, other factors also influence the effectiveness of informal care. These factors—related to the dependent person, to the person giving care, and to the relationship between caregiver and care receiver—both promote caregiving and create barriers. They help explain why a person like Ms. Worth can collect a bevy of surrogate kin helpers, while Mrs. Starr claims few informal ties. In Chapters 6 and 7, we explore in greater detail some of these additional elements that influence both the successes and failures of these elders in getting and keeping the help of family and friends. First, we must lay the groundwork for these discussions by describing each participant's informal caregiving network.

## LUCY OLIVER

Ever since Lucy Oliver had her stroke, her husband of over fifty years has taken care of her. He helps with personal care and does most of the household chores, performing all tasks quite competently. He also arranges for, and accompanies his wife to, her frequent clinic visits and assists with her medications. Mrs. Oliver affirms his primary caregiving role:

> If it wasn't for him, I don't know what I'd do. As long as I been sick, he hardly ever be gone. He do everything here that need to be done.

A few necessary tasks, however, Mr. Oliver cannot do such as plaiting his wife's hair or writing the household checks. Because he no longer has a car, he is not able to provide transportation to the doctor or for more strictly social outings. His limited knowledge of, and sometimes resistance to, conventional health care also restricts his help in these areas.

Although the Olivers' eight children do not provide regular, basic care, some visit, provide emergency assistance, and sporadically furnish other services. Occasionally, one takes their mother shopping, assists with her personal care, or stays with her while Mr. Oliver attends church, an important aspect of his life as a lay minister. Her children's neglect weighs heavily on Mrs. Oliver:

> That's the one thing I get worried about—is having somebody to do something for me. I'm so used to being together. They come by here all the time when I first got sick, and now they don't do it. I say I guess they got tired, but they do anything I tell them. If I get sick or feel bad and call, they'll be over here. As long as I'm doing all right they don't come. Anything I want they're here, but they don't come as often as I think they should come. They'll come to take me to the store. They'll come and see about me if I call. I have enough of them to come by here every day. That's what's the matter with me.

While Mr. Oliver recognizes the responsibilities their children have to their own lives, he confirms the limited care they provide:

They don't hardly help. Some don't even call, as many as they are. I don't know what you have children for. She's been sick for five years. They know she's sick. They know she doesn't like to stay by herself. She thinks somebody can be 'round all the time. People have other things to do. When a child gets grown, have to let go.

Although dedicated and committed to his wife's care, he, too, often experiences stress from his never-ending duties. He has had to give up his informal taxi service and especially misses his regular church activities:

I promised the good Lord I would take care of her as long as I was able, but anybody has to get out sometime. Church is more than on Sunday. Most of the time only time I can rest is when she's gone. Last few days she's just layin' around callin' me every few minutes. I think she's just in the habit of callin'. Stays up all night, every night. I have to stay with her. Don't get a chance to go nowhere.

## RUBY WASHINGTON

Ruby Washington has two primary caregivers—her common-law husband, Mr. Jones, and her son Robert, who lives in the other side of her house. Even before he moved in with her, Mr. Jones came over everyday to help. He now takes care of many basic needs, such as bringing her water for bathing, helping her to dress, doing laundry, cleaning, shopping, and cooking. He pushes her in her wheelchair to church, accompanies her to County for her clinic appointments, helps her walk, and reminds her about her medicine. One time when the first author supplied the transportation for a shopping expedition, he helped pick out Mrs. Washington's new outfit for Easter Sunday. Mr. Jones is committed to caring for his wife, and it is on his care that she depends.

Mrs. Washington's son Robert tends to business matters, such as getting his mother's checks cashed, paying bills, and handling her food stamps. Occasionally he prepares meals. Before his car broke down, he sometimes provided transportation for her and Mr. Jones. Mrs. Washington is confident that Robert will stick by her, but like the Olivers, she feels that he could do more:

Robert hang right to me, but he always got something to do. I get in behind him. Children don't do nothing much. He don't stay here much, out and gone.

Both Robert and Mr. Jones collect Social Security disability and are unemployed. Unlike Mr. Oliver, they are not overwhelmed by their caregiving roles. They both drink regularly, especially around the first of the month when checks arrive, a habit that hinders their effectiveness. Recently Robert was in the county jail for a month for shooting his twenty-three year-old girlfriend in the leg. Mrs. Washington reported that when Robert tried to "quit her," she slashed the tires on his car and threw rocks at the house. During the time Robert was in jail, Mrs. Washington's house was burglarized in the middle of the night, while Mr. Jones slept soundly on the sofa nearby.

One of Mrs. Washington's children, a daughter, is deceased. Another son and daughter live in Philadelphia. These two children are not available to give basic instrumental care, yet they often urge their mother to come live with them, and they do visit at least annually, call regularly, and occasionally send money.

Mrs. Washington has numerous other relatives and friends who provide small services and emotional support. John, a retarded man who lives in the neighborhood, comes by each day and is an ever-willing candidate to make a trip to the corner store or empty the bedpan. One grandson, David, visits daily, and another young man, who lives nearby and calls her "grandma," stops in regularly. Her cousin, Belle, a neighbor and close friend, also quite elderly, frequently sends over food. Another friend, Sallie Mae, calls each night to check on her. Mrs. Washington's church helps in emergencies, as when her money was stolen, and members call or visit and give her small gifts at Christmas.

Mrs. Washington's remaining two sisters and one brother are in poor health themselves, but the siblings keep each other company through frequent phone calls.

With her large network of informal support, most of Mrs. Washington's physical needs are met. She is never lonely or alone.

## ELOISE LITTLE

Unlike the two married women, Eloise Little has no informal caregivers to provide her with basic physical care on a daily basis or to manage her care. Mr. Avant, her roomer, is generally at home, but some days he only turns on her TV and unlocks the front door, for others who might come in. Other days he might prepare food or bring her some fresh water. If asked, he usually consents to a trip to the neighborhood store to pick up a few items, and he regularly pays the household bills. Yet, his manner is often curt and unpleasant.

Even though Mr. Avant plays a minor role in Mrs. Little's day-to-day care, he is available when emergencies arise. One night he rescued Mrs. Little from a rat that had crawled inside her nightgown. Because of her vulnerability, she is thankful for his presence, but sometimes she hesitates to seek his help:

> Mr. Avant will do for me if he know I need it. I'm waiting on him now to come through here to ask him to cook me some steak. I thank him for everything he do. He realize I can't do no walking. I got a bell to call him. He jumps. I try not to worry him. He may not mind, but it's the way he speaks. He talks to me so hateful. Sometimes I do without water all day long. My feelings are easily hurt. I ain't used to anybody talking to me like that. I appreciate him being here with me. Anything could come in here and carry me off, kill me. They think I have money.

Mrs. Little's half-sister, Gertrude, who works full-time, living-in and taking care of an old, impaired white lady, provides only limited, intermittent care. She occasionally comes over to wash clothes, clean up, or work in the yard. More often her visits are brief, typically to drop off some cooked food. If Gertrude happens to be visiting when Mrs. Little needs washing after a bowel or bladder accident, she will help, but this kind of service is rarely given. At times a month will pass without a visit. Mrs. Little neither counts on Gertrude, nor trusts her:

> Gertrude claimed she would do this and do that and wouldn't have time, she and my sister-in-law both. I have to beg them to get those pads [for her bed]. She would cash my check and wouldn't bring back the money, wouldn't half pay the bills.

Mrs. Little's half-brother, Tom, has a car and generally can be depended on to go to County to get her medicine and the pads she needs for her bed. While his wife, Marion, used to wash for Mrs. Little and cash her check, Marion's care now is neither consistent nor extensive. She spends her free time taking care of her grandchildren or going to church, as Mrs. Little noted with some cynicism:

> Marion said she'd be at church all weekend and if anything [i.e., food] left, she'd bring me something. You know how [the] sanctified are—"satisfied."

For awhile Mrs. Little's nephew, Eugene, hung around her house a good bit of the time. Unemployed, alcoholic, and homeless, he frequently slept on her sofa or on the front porch. Sometimes Eugene would walk to the neighborhood store, rub his aunt's shoulders with liniment, or cook a meal. She could not, however, count on him for regular care. More recently, conflicts with Mr. Avant and Gertrude have kept Eugene away altogether.

Two neighbors, Miss Fannie and Rosa Mae, both older widows themselves, also give sporadic care. Miss Fannle lives next door and at one time was a primary caregiver. Unfortunately, her health has deteriorated, and she now only comes over when Mrs. Little calls, usually to bring food or to help clean her up after an accident. On Thanksgiving she cooked a turkey Mrs. Little had been given by a neighborhood church. Rosa Mae also used to provide regular, significant care, even sleeping there at night, but when the neighbors began to spread rumors about her drinking and entertaining men in Mrs. Little's house, she abandoned her primary role. Rosa Mae's help now is limited to what Mrs. Little can persuade her to do—going to the store to buy beer, helping her get ready for clinic appointments, and providing some personal care. Mrs. Little laments the decline in her friends' caregiving services:

> One day I went out on the porch for two hours, and my friend Rosa Mae passed by and didn't even say a word. All at once she quit coming. She always had some excuse; couldn't get Rosa Mae down here. I wanted some water so bad.

> It look like Miss Fannie don't want to fool with me no more. I took Miss Fannie and her sister like kin.

### REVEREND JOSEPH SCOTT

Widowed, with no children, Rev. Scott has few informal helpers and no regular family care. His one brother comes about every three months, to cut his toenails, or when Rev. Scott has special needs, such as when he came home from the hospital. His niece, whom he helped raise, also rarely visits and gives no routine care. Rev. Scott:

> Well, I call on my brother sometimes. He hardly has time, but if it's something he can do on the weekends, he might do that. When I came out of the hospital, he came over and brought a couple of dinners; he came back yesterday and brought me a dinner, barbecue stuff, enough for a couple of days. Couple of times I called on my niece to pick up a few things.

Rev. Scott has four older sisters. The only one in town lives in a nursing home. They all get together on Thanksgiving when his two sisters from the northeast make their annual visits, and they telephone him regularly and send cards or gifts when he is in the hospital.

Rev. Scott's only regular helper is his friend, Deacon Pate, ten years his senior. Deacon Pate provides transportation to medical appointments and church, makes bank deposits, and helps out whenever he can:

> He takes me to church, takes me to the clinic, runs errands for me when I need him to. When he took me to the doctor Friday, he went by to get some office supplies, and this morning he came by and got my automobile tag. He's doing things for me all the time. He put the tag on after he got back. Sometime a little something go wrong with the car, he'll fix that.

Deacon Pate is not available to help, however, on a daily basis with personal care or household tasks, and recently when his wife was sick, he had to discontinue his help for several months. Rev. Scott has no informal support to assist with his daily needs and, as we saw in the preceding chapter, few friends and visitors.

## GERALDINE STARR

Geraldine Starr has lived alone since she left her third husband shortly before he died twelve years ago. She talks on the telephone sometimes to her second husband, but he has heart trouble, and she says, "there's nothing neither one of us can do now for each other." She cannot locate her own two sons from her first marriage (her third son is deceased) and has no contact with any of her step-children from her subsequent unions.

The only family members with whom Mrs. Starr maintains ties are a cousin by marriage, Ethel, and another cousin, Dorothy, on her mother's side of the family. Ethel used to visit regularly, often every Sunday, bringing groceries and cooking meals, enough to last for several days. Now Ethel is herself impaired, with severe rheumatoid arthritis, and recently fell, breaking her hip. Mrs. Starr appreciated, yet sometimes discouraged, Ethel's help:

> Ethel does a lot to be in the shape she's in. She's as sweet to me as she can be. You can look at her hands and see what bad shape she's in, been operated on three times. I don't want her to come all the time.

Her other cousin, Dorothy, rarely visits but will occasionally pick up Mrs. Starr's urinary pads from the pharmacy. She assumed the role of family contact during Mrs. Starr's nursing home stay, and she and her

husband have helped in emergency situations, once even coming to
Mrs. Starr's rescue after a fall in the middle of the night.

Mrs. Starr has two friends that provide some help. Scott, a young
man who teaches music at a local college, infrequently brings her a
meal or some item she needs and once took her out shopping. Her
customer service representative at the bank, Annette, sometimes
provides occasional services. Recently, since Mrs. Starr has become
unable to go to the bank, Annette has filled out the money orders for
her bills and brought cash to her at home. Mrs. Starr receives no
support from other highrise residents.

Mrs. Starr, therefore, has few family and friends to help with her
day-to-day personal needs and frequently proclaims her solitary state:

> I just depend on myself and God almighty.

## VIOLA WORTH

Like Mrs. Starr, Viola Worth is an only child, is estranged from her
son, and has no blood relatives who provide regular care. She does,
however, have a "play family," who take care of many of her instrumental needs. Her goddaughter, Maxine, pays her bills, either takes her
shopping or brings her groceries, and sometimes provides other needed
transportation. A variety of other play children and church members
call with offers of help, bring presents at Christmas and on Mother's
Day, and vie for her presence at their Thanksgiving tables. She and her
play sister enjoy daily telephone visits, and one play son, Leonard, who
lives close by, takes her each month to pick up her check at the post
office and to get it cashed and is available to run short errands. Her
church gives her $30 each month.

Despite their willingness to help, all of Ms. Worth's adopted
family members work full-time and have families of their own.
None can assist regularly with her bath or routine housekeeping
chores or always be available to provide transportation to her doctor or
to get her medicine. At times, several days go by when she has no
visitors and is alone. Nevertheless, she believes they fulfill her most
critical needs and is confident she can depend on them:

> I say there's nothing to it. Just when I need favors, they take me.
> When I want to go to church, they carry me to church. They may
> run errands or take me out to shopping, any little thing that I want
> to get out to I do, 'cause I can't get out on my own. I can even call
> my church. Like I want to go to church, I can call out there. Maxine
> and them do what they can, but I got more than just ya'll and

members. I can call the church and let them send somebody else here. I got somebody whether it's my God-family, play children, or what. I ain't going to tell nobody that maybe I don't get sad and blue sometimes. Maybe my friends, or family as I calls them, maybe they be away a week or two, or sometime I don't hear from them in several days or a week, but I'm supposed to be able to push that off and don't worry about it 'cause everybody got problems of they own. They got business to tend to. As long as you know a person, you feel in their heart they love you or they'd come to your call if you need them, that's the main thing. That's what parents counts, isn't it? Well it means a lot.

### SALLY FINCH

Unlike Ms. Worth, Sally Finch has minimal informal support. One regular helper is her sister-in-law, Faye, who does her grocery shopping once a month and cashes her checks. Faye has health problems herself, however, and no longer takes Mrs. Finch with her to shop because she is not able to lift the wheelchair. Recently, Faye was sick and could not do the monthly shopping. Although Mrs. Finch had a friend that used to shop for her, she no longer trusts her and believes that her sister-in-law is her only alternative:

> I married her brother. She cashes my check and gets groceries once a month. That's the only time I can get it. She done it for two years. About the only one I can trust. Had another girlfriend of mine, I *thought* she was a friend. I found out. She would take the fresh and give me the old. Don't let her handle my money. She would cash my check; spent $15 out of it. If she had just once *asked* me. Never could find the slips. Some people think 'cause you're old, you're a fool. Good way to mess up a friendship—mess with money. I'd let you have it but don't *take* it.

Mrs. Finch was one of eight children, but her only living sister is eighty years old and "down too." The two sisters talk daily on the telephone but only get together when their nephew brings the older sister to Mrs. Finch's apartment, about twice a year. The nephew provides no other help to Mrs. Finch. Neither do her other relatives:

> I have a heap of people, but some of them ain't never seen me; some I've never seen. I have cousins right here in Atlanta never come to see me. Nieces and nephews don't have time. Sometime I don't feel like they're kin to me.

Another resident in the highrise, whom she calls "Doright," is her most frequent helper. He makes purchases for her from the vegetable truck that makes weekly visits to the highrise and takes her cans and bottles to the trash whenever she asks. The lady who lives next door has helped in emergencies when she was sick and had to go to the hospital, and friends from her old neighborhood, John and Ertha, will sometimes get her medicine and on rare occasions accompany her to the clinic.

Although Mrs. Finch can manage a number of instrumental tasks independently, she has no informal caregiver to help with her bath, do the heavy cleaning and laundry, or accompany her regularly to her clinic appointments. She is often alone.

*   *   *   *

Among these participants the availability of informal helpers and the assistance they provide varies greatly. Despite the level of informal care received, each person has needs that are not met by available informal support. These residual needs range from maximum, for Eloise Little, to the minimal needs of Sally Finch and Ruby Washington. Because Mrs. Little has both severe need and little informal support, she needs additional care on a daily basis. In other situations, needs are less critical. Geraldine Starr needs help with cooking, but she can get around her apartment and do some food preparation—even if only preparing a bowl of cereal—and routinely has her groceries delivered. Similarly, when Mrs. Finch has no one to help with her shower, she can wash off at the bathroom sink. Other individuals with minimal informal support are able to perform particular chores on an infrequent basis, though sustained efforts are too burdensome. This is true of Rev. Scott, who, when unassisted, requires most of a day to complete his personal care and meal preparation. Needs for additional help run the gamut from periodic assistance to make life a little better and a little easier to extensive care that provides basic subsistence.

In the two chapters that follow we examine traits of both care receivers and caregivers that influence the informal caregiving relationship and the level of care these helpers provide. In Part III, we explore the capacity of the formal care system to fill these gaps.

## REFERENCES

1. M. Cantor, Families: A Basic Source of Long-term Care for the Elderly, *Aging, 349,* pp. 8-13, 1985.

2. M. Cantor, Neighbors and Friends: An Overlooked Resource in Informal Support System, *Research on Aging, 1*:4, pp. 434-463, 1979.
3. L. R. Fischer, L. Rogne, and N. N. Eustis, Support Systems for the Family-less Elderly: Care Without Commitment, in *Home Care Experience*, J. F. Gubrium and A. Sankar (eds.), Sage Publications, Inc., Newbury Park, California, 1990.
4. J. Morris and S. Sherwood, Informal Support Resources for Vulnerable Elderly Persons: Can They Be Counted On, Why Do They Work?, *International Journal of Aging and Human Development, 18*, pp. 81-98, 1984.
5. E. Stoller and L. Earl, Help with Activities of Everyday Life: Sources of Support for the Noninstitutionalized Elderly, *The Gerontologist, 23*, pp. 64-69, 1983.
6. S. J. Brody, W. Poulshock, and C. F. Musciocchi, The Family Caring Unit: A Major Consideration in the Long-term Support System, *The Gerontologist, 18*, pp. 556-561, 1978.
7. E. Shanas, Social Myth as Hypothesis: The Case of Family Relations of Old People, *The Gerontologist, 19*, pp. 3-9, 1979.
8. T. Wan and W. Weissert, Social Support Networks, Patient Status and Institutionalization, *Research on Aging, 3*, pp. 240-256, 1981.
9. A. M. Jette, L. G. Branch, L. A. Sleeper, H. Feldman, and L. M. Sullivan, High-Risk Profiles for Nursing Home Admission, *The Gerontologist, 32*:5, pp. 635-640, 1992.
10. C. L. Johnson, Dyadic Family Relations and Social Support, *The Gerontologist, 23*, pp. 377-383, 1983.
11. L. M. Chatters, R. J. Jackson, and J. S. Jackson, Aged Blacks' Choices for an Informal Helper Network, *Journal of Gerontology, 41*:1, pp. 94-100, 1986.
12. R. C. Gibson and J. S. Jackson, The Health, Physical Functioning, and Informal Supports of the Black Elderly, *The Milbank Quarterly, 65*, pp. 421-454, 1987.
13. M. Cantor, Strain Among Caregivers: A Study of Experience in the United States, *The Gerontologist, 21*, pp. 597-604, 1983.
14. C. L. Johnson and D. J. Catalano, Childless Elderly and Their Family Supports, *The Gerontologist, 21*, pp. 610-618, 1981.
15. C. L. Johnson and D. J. Catalano, A Longitudinal Study of Family Supports to the Impaired Elderly, *The Gerontologist, 23*, pp. 612-618, 1983.
16. E. Stoller, Parental Caregiving by Adult Children, *Journal of Marriage and the Family, 45*, pp. 851-858, 1983.
17. L. Crossman, C. London, and C. Barry, Older Women Caring for Disabled Spouses: A Model for Supportive Services, *The Gerontologist, 21*, pp. 464-470, 1981.
18. K. Jonas and E. Wellin, Dependency and Reciprocity: Home Health Aid in an Elderly Population, in *Aging in Culture and Society: Comparative Viewpoints and Strategies*, C. Fry (ed.), J. F. Bergin, Brooklyn, 1980.

19. E. K. Abel, Daughters Caring for Elderly Parents, in *The Home Care Experience*, J. F. Gubrium and A. Sankar (eds.), Sage Publications, Inc., Newbury Park, California, 1990.
20. J. Morris and S. Sherwood, Informal Support Resources for Vulnerable Elderly Persons: Can They Be Counted On, Why Do They Work? *International Journal of Aging and Human Development, 18*, pp. 81-98, 1984.
21. B. Robinson and M. Thurnher, Taking Care of Aged Parents, *The Gerontologist, 19*, pp. 586-593, 1979.
22. J. Scott, Siblings and Other Kin, in *Family Relations in Later Life*, T. H. Brubaker (ed.), Sage Publications, Inc., Beverly Hills, California, 1983.
23. G. J. Wentowski, Reciprocity and the Coping Strategies of Older People: Cultural Dimensions of Network Building, *The Gerontologist, 21*, pp. 600-609, 1981.
24. L. R. Hatch, Informal Support Patterns of Older African-American and White Women, *Research on Aging, 13*:2, pp. 144-170, June 1991.
25. J. J. Jackson, *Minorities and Aging*, Wadsworth Publishing Co., Belmont, California, 1980.
26. C. L. Johnson and B. Barer, Families and Networks among Older Inner-City Blacks, *The Gerontologist, 30*, pp. 726-733, 1990.
27 J. Mitchell and J. C. Regis
   the Elderly by Race, Socioeconomic Status and Residence, *The Gerontologist, 24*, pp. 48-54, 1984.
28. E. Mutran, Intergenerational Family Support among Blacks and Whites: Response to Culture or to Socioeconomic Differences, *Journal of Gerontology, 40*:3, pp. 382-389, 1985.
29. C. Stack, *All Our Kin*, Harper and Row, New York, 1974.
30. C. G. Wenger, Personal Care: Variations in Network Type, Style, and Capacity, in *The Home Care Experience*, J. F. Gubrium and A. Sankar (eds.), Sage Publications, Inc., Newbury Park, California, 1990.
31. C. L. Johnson and L. E. Troll, Constraints and Facilitators to Friendships in Late Late Life, *The Gerontologist, 34*:1, pp. 79-87, 1994.
32. J. C. Barker and L. S. Mitteness, Invisible Caregivers in the Spotlight: Non-kin Caregivers of Frail Older Adults, in *The Home Care Experience*, J. F. Gubrium and A. Sankar (eds.), Sage Publications, Inc., Newbury Park, California, 1990.
33. N. Rosel, The Hub of a Wheel: A Neighborhood Support Network, *International Journal of Aging and Human Development, 16*, pp. 193-200, 1983.
34. S. Sherman, Mutual Assistance and Support in Retirement Housing, *Journal of Gerontology, 30*, pp. 479-483, 1975.
35. J. Smithers, *Determined Survivors: Community Life among the Urban Elderly*, Rutgers University Press, New Brunswick, New Jersey, 1985.
36. L. R. Fischer, L. Rogne, and N. N. Eustis, Support Systems for the Familyless Elderly: Care Without Commitment, in *The Home Care Experience*, J. F. Gubrium and A. Sankar (eds.), Sage Publications, Inc., Newbury Park, California, 1990.

37. D. T. Gold, Late-life Sibling Relationships: Does Race Affect Typological Distribution? *The Gerontologist, 30*:6, p. 5, 1990.
38. C. T. Walls and S. H. Zarit, Informal Support from Black Churches and the Well-Being of Elderly Blacks, *The Gerontologist, 31*:4, pp. 490-495, 1991.
39. S. A. Lockery, Family and Social Supports: Caregiving among Racial and Ethnic Minority Elders, *Generations, XV*:1, pp. 58-62, 1991.
40. M. B. Sussman, The Family Life of Old People, in *Handbook of Aging and the Social Sciences,* R. H. Binstock and E. Shanas (eds.), Van Nostrand Reinhold, New York, pp. 218-243, 1976.
41. K. R. Allen, and V. Chin-Sang, A Lifetime of Work: The Context and Meanings of Leisure for Aging Black Women, *The Gerontologist, 30*:1 pp. 734-740, 1990.
42. R. L. Rubinstein, B. B. Alexander, M. Goodman, and M. Luborsky, Key Relationships of Never Married, Childless Older Women: A Cultural Analysis, *Journal of Gerontology: Social Sciences, 46*:5, pp. S270-S277, 1991 .
43. S. I. White-Means, Informal Home Care for Frail Black Elderly, *Journal of Applied Gerontology, 12*:1, pp. 13-33, March 1993.

# CHAPTER
# 6

# The Dilemma of Dependency

*Sometimes I may be too independent, but I thank God for my little independence. Just don't let me get where I can't do nothing for myself and keep me with my stout [strength] where I can stir around a little bit. When I get worser where they have to stick them needles in me, take me on home from here [let me die] 'cause I didn't come here to stay.*

Viola Worth

*Oh, I didn't know it was going to be so hard. Can't get out. Have to depend on somebody else to do. I have a hard time. I know if you get older, you're gonna hurt. Just have to depend on other people. That's the hardest part. I worry about that. Look like nobody care about you: living, but look like you in somebody else's way. You know, it's just hard.*

Sally Finch

The words of Viola Worth, who is still independent in many ways, express the preference for independence that each of these seven African American elders share. In Chapter 2, we saw day-to-day evidence that, despite significant disability and often with considerable effort, they try to take care of their own basic needs. Even small successes brought satisfaction, while the inability to accomplish necessary tasks independently often causes frustration, anger, and despair.

Dependency is the other side of the coin—in Sally Finch's view, "the hardest part." The emotions related to being dependent, to feeling burdensome, useless, and without power, intensify the value of autonomy.

Such attitudes espousing independence are not unique among older persons. Independence is a personal goal widespread in American culture, and evidence is convincing that this value does not fade as people age or become disabled [1-5]. Brian Hofland has described three dimensions of autonomy: 1) physical, which relates to freedom of mobility and physical independence, 2) psychological, relating to control over one's environment and to choice of options, and 3) spiritual, which involves an expanded concept of self and relates to a continuity in the sense of personal identity over time [5]. The reality of life for these seven elders is a loss of autonomy in each of these dimensions. The value for autonomy remains firm, but it takes on new meaning, even as it ebbs.

The meanings people attach to independence and dependence significantly influence behaviors related to receiving care. They help explain why some people with little social support still resist assistance, and others with extensive support systems continue to have unmet needs. The help that caregivers provide frequently impinges on the very freedom and independence that frail elderly persons value, creating tensions in the caregiving situation—between the self-determination of the dependent person and the decisions and standards of the caregiver [6]. Caregivers often feel forced to choose between respecting a person's autonomy on one hand while promoting the person's well-being on the other. Collopy suggests that this choice "is nettled with dilemma, since it requires not simply choosing right from wrong, but choosing right from right, choosing one value over another" [7, p. 9].

The caregiving process can become a struggle for power between a well-meaning caregiver and a recalcitrant recipient. Such struggles are a regular occurrence in nursing homes, where a resident's right to self-determination has been mandated by law. The Nursing Home Reform Act of 1987 gives residents the right to make their own decisions about the care they receive, including the right to make what many caregivers believe to be "bad" choices. Studies that have examined the perspective of nursing home residents clearly demonstrate that possessing this decisional capacity is of vital importance to them [8].

In this chapter we examine these attitudes and feelings that are so central to these seven African Americans, as they are to many individuals who can no longer provide for their own basic needs. The data suggest two fundamental and interrelated elements make up the value for independence: 1) maintaining an independent identity and 2) maintaining control over one's life. For these elders with declining resources, this value often cannot be realized to the degree desired, but it is never abandoned. We see that strategies are developed to attain this valued status to the greatest extent possible, even though these strategies may mean negotiating only an appearance of greater independence or stretching one's values.

## THE ROOTS OF INDEPENDENCE

The feelings and emotions that people have about dependency are filtered through their life experiences and personalities. The self-reliance professed by Ms. Worth is rooted in a self-proclaimed toughness developed early in life:

> I've been a tough jack all my life. Not bad, just sticking up for myself.

Her mother died when she was six, and she was raised by her "auntie" until she left home in her teens. In many ways she has had to fend for herself since then, never marrying and living on her own or with whatever white family employed her. Each of these seven elders has experienced tough times, and each has been accustomed to taking care of his or her own needs and often the needs of others as well. They belong to the cohort brought up in the early 1900s, a group known to hold dear their independence [9]. One study of older black women suggests that lifetimes of adversity, such as these elders have experienced, encourage the development of psychological and social strengths that lead to self-reliance in old age [10]. For Geraldine Starr, the wellspring of her stubborn independence can be traced to her history:

> I'm used to standing on myself. I try not to depend on people. I never dreamed I'd get down where I couldn't do for myself. I'm used to waitin' on other people. Got to learn to vouch for yourself.

Despite an ideology that values independence, the real world of these participants often is of ever-increasing dependence, and, for some, the ensuing angst is only sharpened by these memories of their former lives in which they were fully independent people accustomed to "doing." When Mrs. Finch measures the present against her past life of hard work, it comes up short. Even though her life now is more comfortable and economically secure than at any other time, her satisfaction is tempered because she no longer can do for herself the little everyday things she has always done—the things most people take for granted:

Have been hard times. I worked but I wasn't making anything. It's good now, but it's tough when you can't get out and do for yourself, especially when you're used to doing and get where you can't. Some people never did anything anyway.

Even Ms. Worth, usually upbeat and still proud of her daily successes, sometimes is despondent over her lack of independence:

Worrying can kill you. Joyful as I try to be, I get depressed too. That's the way it is when you can't do nothing for yourself. Mind will get to traveling, least little something. . . .

For some of the elders described here, a lifetime of independence includes a reluctance to form interdependent ties with others. Mrs. Starr, as we saw in Chapter 4, does not associate with her neighbors in the highrise; nor does she depend on them for support. For her, this self-reliant behavior too has been a lifelong pattern:

I don't loan nothing to nobody and I don't borrow nothing from nobody. My mother didn't either. I just wasn't brought up to lean on somebody else. Maybe I have the wrong attitude.

Eloise Little is quick to explain that her parallel behavior does not represent selfishness, but, instead, embodies the culture she was taught:

I didn't ask nobody for nothing; never been that way. I was raised up that way. I ain't gonna borrow. You bought it for your use. I bought it for my use. I wouldn't borrow salt, sugar, or coffee. If I didn't have it, I would wait till I could get it. Couldn't borrow from me either. Couldn't call me selfish. That's the way I was brought up.

Clearly, such life-long traditions of "standing on one's own" encourage neither requesting nor accepting help.

## STAYING IN CONTROL

Central to the dilemma of dependency is the fear of losing control over one's personal life. This desire to retain control is a significant factor in the decisions of these individuals to remain in their own homes. Mrs. Little has been urged by both formal and informal caregivers to re-enter a nursing home, but strongly resists such advice, even at the risk of significant deprivation. The foremost reason guiding her resistance is her desire to retain control—to be her own "boss":

> I don't want to be in no home at all. I want to be in my own home. Don't want nobody bossin' me around.

Mrs. Starr, who also has had an unsatisfactory nursing home experience, voices similar concerns about having to give up the right to make day-to-day choices:

> They want to treat these old people like children. I'm an old grey woman. Don't try to tell me what to put on. . . . Have to eat the same thing everyday. Get so sick of grits and eggs. We had a big blowout about my wanting a piece of ham. I got it too.

Most older people do not have to experience nursing home life firsthand to conceive the grim imagery. Just visiting a friend or hearing the horror stories that abound often is sufficient to engender an enduring fear. Ms. Worth has a vivid mental picture and is adamant that nursing home placement would be her last resort. For her too, apprehension centers around the potential loss of ability to make life's ordinary choices:

> I pictures that time I [might] go in a nursing home—I got to wait till they say I can eat. I got my junk [at home], I can go in there and eat what I want to or pick up what I want. Can't have nothing in your room but certain stuff. Some of these nursing homes don't even let 'em catch no air [go outside]; maybe get out in the lobby sometime. I'm gonna leave ya'll right here. I don't think I would last long if I was just forced to do that because when you done lived by yourself, or done done like you want all your life, it's something about it. It changes you. Well, I tell you I ain't crazy. You may think I'm crazy but I'd rather for God to take me than to have to go anywhere. When he say you got to go, I say, "O.K., Jesus just take me on with you."

These same concerns about autonomy and choice influence decisions about moving into the home of a caregiver. Ruby Washington refuses to go to Philadelphia to live in her daughter's home. Although she now shares her home with her son, it is still *her* home:

> I don't want to live with no one. If my grandson built me my own house, I might go.

With parallel motivation, Mrs. Starr rejected the offer of an aide at the nursing home of a place in her own home:

> Why? So you can boss me around? I just don't want it. I'd rather try to fight it out myself.

Other research corroborates the passion of these informants to remain in their own homes rather than share the homes of others or enter an institution [4, 11]. The qualitative works of Gubrium [12] and Rubinstein and colleagues [3] validate that motives related to control and choice largely govern these preferences.

While giving up one's home can represent the ultimate loss of control, control over one's life also diminishes with each lost capacity to accomplish tasks necessary for daily living. Loss of control translates into loss of freedom to do what one wants, when and how one wants to, and this loss is extremely troubling to each of these individuals. As Kaufman suggested in her study of the sources of meaning in old age, the meaningfulness of daily life depends not on what people do, but on the ability to choose [13].

The loss of control inherent in a dependent situation represents a loss of power relative to those who provide the needed care. As we see in the following chapter, the reluctance to relinquish power—and ultimately control—to the caregiver has significant impact on the care relationship. It influences both the strategies used to get help and the continuing efforts to get by without it. The desire for control influences Mrs. Little's decision not to let her half-sister Gertrude manage her money, even though Mrs. Little herself has difficulty performing this task and sometimes even loses her scarce funds. The rationale governing her behavior emerges from an assessment of Gertrude that has developed over the historical course of their interactions—that is, if Gertrude has control of her money, she will then try to tell her how to spend it and, more importantly, will not let her "drink it up." Preserving control motivates Mrs. Starr to order her groceries over the phone rather than asking someone to shop for her. Although her first choice would be to go to the store herself to pick out the groceries she wants, the next best available alternative—the one that gives her the most control—is having them delivered, when she "has a taste for them," rather than at the convenience of a caregiver.

We also see that the desire for control extends to control of personal space, no matter how constricted this space may become. Eloise Little tries desperately to hold out against her family's attempts to clean up her room. Preserving her reduced personal environment, holding on to her things, is infinitely more important to her than the clean and tidy space her family would prefer:

> I don't like for folks to go in my things when I told 'em what I was saving 'em for. I've had so many things taken from me. I had all the things an old woman could want. I'm gonna have this rabbit, basket, and flower [some trinkets people had given her] till funeral day.

These "things" she speaks of are on her bed and thereby within her realm of control. Rubinstein and colleagues discovered similar attempts by impaired elders to retain control of their reduced personal environments, which may even become expressions of themselves [3]. While Mrs. Little's things may seem insignificant to her caregivers, they are things she can arrange and sort out, giving her something to do and be—another role and identity—besides a compliant old woman.

## MANAGING IDENTITIES

Increased disability and the ensuing dependency represent more than just loss of power. Also lost are many of the former roles of a productive life. Although role loss is common in old age because of such factors as retirement and death of one's family and friends [14, 15], functional impairment obviously compounds the problem. Of these seven participants, only Rev. Scott is able to perform a traditional work role, and its scope is limited. Social roles also are reduced significantly. Except for Mrs. Oliver and Mrs. Washington, who have husbands and children, they no longer can claim the role of spouse or parent, and only in limited circumstances can they act as friends.

Roles help people define their identity. Identity theory [16] emphasizes the capacity of humans to create and use symbols in interactions with each other [17]. It is through social interactions that we construct our own social reality and sense of self. Humans are not passive observers of situations, rather we react to our surroundings. Through interpreting and evaluating the meanings of our interactions with others, we define each situation and use the resulting definition to organize our own behavior.

The tenets of identity theory stem also from William James's contention that people have as many identities as the number of distinct sets of structured relationships in which they are involved [18]. Identities are not valued equally, and identity salience refers to the hierarchal ordering of these identities. The probability of a particular identity being evoked depends on the defining characteristics of the situation and certain characteristics of self, such as self-esteem or satisfaction.

With few options for performing valued roles, few sets of others with whom to interact, and few situations that allow alternative identities to be expressed, these individuals strive to hold on to some identity other than that of an impaired, dependent person, a person who needs care. Yet, as we discussed in Chapter 3, it is often the less salient identities they evoke. Each person identifies herself/himself as sick and to a greater or lesser degree has adopted the sick role. Mrs. Washington refers to herself as a "diabetes person"; Mrs. Little calls herself "half-dead"; Mrs. Starr is "everything excepting dead"; Mrs. Finch is "broke-up"; and Ms. Worth's body is "twisted." These ways of self-identification of course stem from the manifestations of disease and disability, but they have emerged also through interactions with others who view them foremost as stigmatized persons rather than as whole individuals. As Savishinsky noted in his discussion of nursing home residents, social attitudes can disable elderly people as much as illness [19]. Just being stigmatized as old and disabled can lead to further decline.

Goffman discussed how identities become damaged when disabled individuals are stigmatized by their impaired conditions [20]. He emphasized that the effect of the attribute causing the stigmatization depends on the situation—that is, stigma can be seen more as a relationship, a result of a social interaction, than an attribute. Damage occurs when wheelchair patients are made to wait until last at the public hospital, when friends cease to visit, or when church members laugh at a post-stroke speech impediment. It happens in interactions with health care professionals when one is cast in the dependent (subordinate) role of patient, and it happens in interactions with caregivers where one is viewed as burdensome. In contrast, when Lucy Oliver is at the adult day care center amongst her disabled compatriots, she does not feel stigmatized by her halting speech because as she professes, "there's something the matter with all of us here."

Most impaired persons do not want their damaged self to become the keystone of self-definition; nor do they want their impaired self to be considered their entire self [21]. Viola Worth expresses this desire succinctly:

> I been handicapped all my life, and I ain't never wanted to be pitied
> for my condition. The average one [handicapped person] don't want

it. Just look at 'em like a human being like you. I hope I made myself clear. If I'm in my right mind, I'd rather not be pitied 'cause it makes me feel bad. As long as I can feel O.K., I'm all right. I feel like I'm like any of the rest of you—I just can't get out there and do for myself like I once did, but if you want to look at it like that, I ain't *never* been able to do for myself like some of you 'cause I been handicapped all my life, but it haven't held me, it haven't cut my spirit, it haven't made me feel like I'm less than nobody else. We all human and we got a handicap. Some born in worse shape than I was. That's what I mean when I say I don't like pity. Instead of pitying a person, help 'em on their way, just like ya'll are doing.

While Ms. Worth is quick to proclaim her lifelong handicap, she makes equal effort to portray other selves. Like many stigmatized persons, she has tried to develop strategies for repairing her damaged identity. One strategy she uses is to try to define herself as independent—by performing the activities she is still able to do. As we saw in Chapter 2, Ms. Worth takes great pride in what she *can* still do, and in her interactions with others she tries to manage her identity by presenting her independent self:

I just like to do things anyway. I try. That's why I like to stay here by myself. I can get in my chair and start to rolling. I don't worry no one but me, not if I can help it. I got a lot of pride doing by myself. There some things maybe I can do, why worry you? I'm so proud that I can do as well as I do. I know the shape I'm in. I know how I feel, yet still I push myself. Sometime they might see me look like I'm almost crawlin', but I'm not ashamed, and I don't want nobody to say, "poor thing," 'cause I ain't no poor thing: I'm trying to make it by the help of God.

Like the impaired elders described by Rubinstein and colleagues [3, p. 146], Ms. Worth and the other informants try to "maintain the self" through continuing what were probably old activities as well as dignifying necessities. Because of this need to present a more positive identity, even Mrs. Little asserts that she always has something to do even if it's just "straightening out her baskets." Such "stretching" of values has been described by Hyman Rodman as a strategy poor people use to adjust to the circumstances of poverty [22]. In a similar vein Kaufman explains how old people are able to reinterpret experiences to give old values new meaning more appropriate to their present circumstances [13]. In the case of these participants, the value of independence is being stretched to accommodate their impaired abilities. This desire for alternative identities offers additional explanation for their determined efforts to be self-reliant, even though the value often takes on new meaning.

The desire for independence in performing activities of daily living, does not necessarily apply to all activities in the same way for each individual. Rather, each person strives to hold onto those roles which are most salient and satisfying and which have been most prominent throughout their lives. Most salient for these women are the cooking and housekeeping activities that were the traditional work and family roles of their former lives. Like the African American women in Allen and Chin-Sang's study of the meanings of work and leisure, domestic work for these women represents a life course continuity that dominated both childhood and adulthood [10]. Rev. Scott, on the other hand, would be quite happy never performing the household chores that traditionally were the domain of the women in his family. While he makes the effort to cook or wash dishes when necessary, he prefers to identify himself with the more salient roles of contractor, accountant, or, when the rare occasion permits it, preacher. In her examination of the concept of self in old age, Kaufman emphasized that old people express a continuity of identity that transcends the physical and social changes that accompany aging [13]. We found that our informants also interpret and give meaning to their experiences in the context of their past lives.

Individuals like Lucy Oliver and Eloise Little, who are more significantly impaired, are rarely able to exercise an independent identity, yet they retain a tight grip on the ideal. Mrs. Oliver continues to hope that she will once again be able to perform these tasks, even though her husband is quite willing and able to do them all:

> I hope and pray to the Lord. I know I ain't going to get well, but I want to get more strong where I can do more things. I want to get where I can do little things everyday. I can make my bed, but it makes me tired.

And Mrs. Little still longs for her former role of housekeeper:

> I want to go back in the kitchen and make me some light biscuit bread. I due to be working somewhere. I sure wish I could go. Want the water, can't get the water. It's kind of hard for me to want to do something and can't do it. There's somebody pitying me.

Sometimes an individual tries to negotiate his or her identity or re-define a situation to give the impression of greater independence—a strategy labeled "impression management" by Goffman [23] and discussed by Matthews [24] in her study of older women. When Ms. Worth pays her bills, she places the exact amount of money needed for each bill in a stamped and addressed envelope, but she still needs a helper to take her to the post office to get her checks and to the liquor store to get them cashed and then to write the checks for each bill. Yet, in her mind, *she* pays the bills, as she explains:

> As far as I'm concerned, when I see what it is and put it in here, I done paid it. These other people write checks. I pay my money. They are paid when I turn 'em over to you. See what I do here—I get my bills, and I do what I'm supposed to do. See, when I give it [the envelopes with the money] to them they ain't got nothing to do but check it out and write the check.

Like the elders described by Rubinstein and colleagues [3] and by Kaufman [13], Ms. Worth has redefined or reinterpreted independence.

For Viola Worth, as for each of these informants, a self-reliant attitude is based also on a realistic appraisal of a situation where no one else may be available to do a needed task. Caregiving arrangements are sometimes precarious, and even with regular helpers, needs are likely to arise that no one is available to meet. The best strategy for some then lies in ever maintaining the effort to do for oneself, Ms. Worth's fervent motto:

> If I sit and hold my fingers and can do, I won't get nowhere. I can't be sitting here when I can do something for myself. What I'm gonna do those days ain't no one around?

The lack of other alternatives created added incentives for Eloise Little to continue her struggles to get herself out of bed without assistance as long as she possibly could. For her refusals of offers to assist with the torturous process, she offered the following explanation:

> I can do it by myself because I'm *here* by myself.

Similar motivations prompted Geraldine Starr to push herself beyond even what she believed was expected of her:

> I press myself too hard. It's not a matter of giving up, trying to 'bate my pains. I should rest, but I ain't got nobody to do.

Wenger found similar high expectations for self-reliance in response to realistic appraisals of support networks among older people in Wales [25].

## BEING HELPED

A common attitude, as expressed by Sally Finch, is that dependent persons are burdensome or "in the way." For Mrs. Finch and for others, these feelings of being burdensome, are supported by the belief that people often do *not* want to help, do *not* want to be bothered. Geraldine Starr frequently lamented the absence of altruism among the human race:

> I asked the Lord to let me suffer on my feet, not flat on my back. Nobody gonna help you when you get flat on your back. Nobody don't want to help. They don't seem to care. Everybody's looking for something. People ain't got time to take up your sympathy and rock it. You got to map that out yourself.

Such attitudes, or ways of defining social reality, often develop through interactions with helpers and would-be helpers. Potential caregivers who mirror a reluctance to help discourage requests, or even acceptance, of needed assistance. Rev. Scott explains how a grudging response prompted him to cease his requests:

> I remember having a young man that used to live here, went off got married, got an apartment. He and his wife used to come see us. After my wife died, I called on him for one or two little things. I called him one day, and he said, "What you want now, Rev?" I took it that he didn't want to be bothered, and I haven't bothered him no more. I just called to see how they were doing. I hadn't heard from them in a pretty good while. He had done things like taking me some place. I hadn't called on him for any money as such. He didn't have time to fool with me, didn't want to be bothered. I just left him alone.

This perception of unwillingness on the part of others prevailed in situations where caregivers were both kin and non-kin. As noted previously, both Mrs. Oliver and Mrs. Washington had children whom they felt did not want to help. In other cases, siblings, nieces, nephews, and cousins were deemed unwilling. Where the caregiver was a spouse, however, a willing commitment to help was acknowledged on both sides.

Ms. Worth, who has numerous helpers but none who provide extensive care, agrees that some people are unwilling to help, but true to her optimistic nature, she looks for the bright side, focusing more on those favorably inclined to provide care. Like Rev. Scott, her experiences have helped define her reality, and she has adjusted her behavior accordingly:

> There are people in this world that don't care too much for me, but that's people's nature. Everybody don't like everybody. If you don't give the opening to be around you, they won't be around you. That's what I call feeding them out of a long handled spoon. Just keep a-lookin' for the best. I don't mind calling nobody and asking them, not if they don't seem to mind doing it. If I get the feeling they trying to drag on it or something, I know I wouldn't call them. Matter of fact when I feel in my heart, practically know you don't care about being bothered with me, I'd rather for you not to come around. So I don't worry about it. There's always going to be somebody out there trying to tear you down, trying to point a finger at you, or wondering about you, but they're feeding it to their ignorance. Just keep a going.

As we saw in Chapter 4, rational decisions often are made to avoid certain threatening social situations [24], those for example that caused embarrassment. The same motivation plays a role in the avoidance of interactions with reluctant helpers. Ms. Worth avoids requesting assistance from people she perceives as unwilling. For her, having to be helped is infinitely more acceptable from an emotional standpoint if a would-be helper's offers of assistance are unsolicited and when requests for help are fulfilled with apparent willingness. This perception not only guides her strategies to get help, but affects her self-image as well:

> Look, you try to help me. You ain't *got* to, ain't nobody *got* to do nothing. See what I'm saying? You ain't got to call me and say, "Do you need anything?" or, "Can I come over and sit with you?" That make me feel *good*. That make me feel like I'm thought of. There's somebody out there cares.

The effect of caregiver reactions on the perceived status of the care receiver was observed by Lustbader [2], a social worker, in relationships between her clients and their informal caregivers as well as by Matthews [24] in her study of old mothers and their children. Lustbader argued that dependent persons, in their inferior and insecure state, begin to look for and anticipate signs of reluctance in the expressions and actions of their helpers and adjust their behavior accordingly [2].

While help freely offered makes Ms. Worth feel cared for, she understands that where need is great neither the giving nor receiving of help is easy:

> I don't have no complaints, because to be a shut-in—be where you can't get around without somebody, can't go nowhere, tend to your business or do things for yourself unlessen somebody have to carry you—I think as happy as I think I'm living and holding my head up, nine years as a shut-in, I think I'm really well taken care of in the spirit of God. You know you can't live in this world by yourself. You have to have somebody. I believe there's a lot of people that have the mind I have [think like I do], rather go on [die] than to be here suffering, leaning on someone. They do what they can for you and all, but everybody got to work. You can't pay nobody's rent. They can't be just sitting up there with you all the time. I don't want nobody here *all* the time. That's what you call a two-way street and being honest about it, that's the way it goes.

For Ms. Worth, being able to depend on her helpers to come when she needs them is more crucial than the greater frequency of care she might also desire. This viewpoint allows her to rationalize the reality of her situation, making it more acceptable:

> I ain't going to tell nobody that maybe I don't get sad and blue sometimes. Maybe my friends, or family as I calls them, maybe they be away a week or two, or sometime I don't hear from them in several days or a week, but I'm supposed to be able to push that off and don't worry about it 'cause everybody got problems of they own. They got business to tend to. As long as you know a person, you feel in their heart they love you or they'd come to your call if you need them, that's the main thing.

As Johnson and Barer discovered in their study of support networks among inner-city blacks, when expectations are lower, disappointments also are lessened [26].

For Lucy Oliver, however, the dependable response of her children to her health crises does not satisfy her. She longs for more attention, despite the many work and family responsibilities they have. Mrs. Oliver's personal history supports the belief that her children should provide the same level of care she once gave to her own mother:

> All of them got children. They have to see after their children. They young, they married, they ain't got time. People don't have time to

do all that. They think about theyself. They can't get self out the way. I know when I used to tend to my mama, I used to work and go home and go to my mama's house and stay to twelve or one o'clock. I didn't get tired. They don't think about getting in the same shape, but they will do for me.

Mrs. Oliver's inability to accept her children's neglect increases her stress and anxiety.

Finally, some people react negatively to being helped simply because they dislike the way a caregiving task is performed. Often what is required for satisfaction is that the task be done the way the dependent person once did it him- or herself. Even Mrs. Little, with few remaining self-care abilities, expressed this notion emphatically:

My way of doing is my best way!

And Mrs. Starr frequently railed against helpers who seemed incapable of following her specifications. Her own high standards only nurtured her resistance to being helped:

I don't like folks fumbling all over me. People can't bathe you like you bathe yourself. Nobody can dress you like you dress yourself. Sometimes I can hardly lift my leg up but I get my shoes on. I ain't gonna give up. My mama was just like that. She wouldn't let nobody fool with her but me. Wait till I can't help myself. That's the way I am. I did that in the hospital. Nobody can't wash my hair like I do. They ain't got time. So I do for myself as long as I can.

* * * * *

In the following chapter, we focus on the behaviors guided by the fundamental value for independence and its two key elements—the staunch desire to preserve autonomy and control and to maintain independent identities. We explore relationships with caregivers, and we examine the strategies these participants use both to get and to resist needed help. These interactions are viewed as exchanges in which recipients "bargain" for the best care "deal" they can get. Additional barriers to providing care also will be discussed, encompassing those inherent in the caregiver's situation (the costs of caregiving) as well as those of the dependent person (the costs of being helped).

# REFERENCES

1. R. P. Abeles, H. G. Gift, and M. G. Ory (eds.), *Aging and Quality of Life: Charting New Territories in Behavioral Science Research*, Springer Publishing Co., New York, 1994.
2. W. Lustbader, *Counting on Kindness: The Dilemmas of Dependency*, The Free Press, New York, 1991.
3. R. L. Rubinstein, J. C. Kilbride, and S. Nagy, *Elders Living Alone*, Aldine de Gruyter, New York, 1992.
4. E. Shanas, Older People and Their Families: The New Pioneers, *Journal of Marriage and the Family, 42*, pp. 9-15, 1980.
5. B. F. Hofland, Why a Special Focus on Autonomy?, *Generations, XIV*:Supplement, pp. 5-8, 1990.
6. B. Collopy, Autonomy in Long Term Care: Some Crucial Distinctions, *The Gerontologist, 28*:Supplement, pp. 10-17, 1988.
7. B. J. Collopy, Ethical Dimensions of Autonomy in Long-Term Care, *Generations, XIV*:Supplement, pp. 9-12, 1990.
8. National Citizens' Coalition for Nursing Home Reform, *A Consumer Perspective on Quality of Care: The Residents' Point of View*, Washington, D.C., 1985.
9. S. E. Levkoff, P. D. Cleary, T. Wetle, and R. W. Besdine, Illness Behavior in the Aged: Implications for Clinicians, *Journal of the American Geriatrics Society, 36*, pp. 622-629, 1988.
10. K. R. Allen and V. Chin-Sang, A Lifetime of Work: The Context and Meanings of Leisure for Aging Black Women, *The Gerontologist, 30*:6, pp. 734-740, 1990.
11. N. Rosel, The Hub of a Wheel: A Neighborhood Support Network, *International Journal of Aging and Human Development, 16*, pp. 193-200, 1983.
12. J. F. Gubrium, *The Mosaic of Care*, Springer, New York, 1991.
13. S. Kaufman, *The Ageless Self: Sources of Meaning in Late Life*, The University of Wisconsin Press, Madison, Wisconsin, 1986.
14. I. Rosow, *Socialization to Old Age*, University of California Press, Berkeley, California, 1974.
15. G. A. Allan and R. G. Adams, Aging and the Structure of Friendship, in *Older Adult Friendships*, R. G. Adams and R. Blieszner (eds.), Sage Publications, Inc., Newbury Park, California, 1989.
16. S. Stryker and R. Serpe, Commitment, Identity Salience, and Role Behavior: Theory and Research Example, in *Personality, Roles, and Social Behavior*, W. Ickes and E. S. Knowles (eds.), Springer-Verlag, New York, pp. 199-218, 1982.
17. R. H. Turner, Unanswered Questions in the Convergence between Structuralist and Interactionist, in *Micro-Theory*, H. J. Helle and S. N. Eisenstadt (eds.), Vol. 2, Sage Publications, Inc., London, 1985.
18. W. James, The Self, *The Principles of Psychology*, Henry Holt, New York, pp. 292-299, 1896.

19. J. Savishinsky, *The Ends of Time: Life and Work in a Nursing Home*, Bergin and Garvey, New York, 1991.
20. E. Goffman, *Stigma: Notes on Management of Spoiled Identity*, Prentice Hall, Englewood Cliffs, New Jersey, 1963.
21. T. E. Levitan, Deviants as Active Participants in the Labeling Process: The Visibly Handicapped, *Social Problems, 22*, pp. 548-557, 1975.
22. H. Rodman, *Lower Class Families: The Culture of Poverty in Negro Trinidad*, Oxford University Press, New York, 1971.
23. E. Goffman, *The Presentation of Self in Everyday Life*, Anchor Books, New York, 1959.
24. S. Matthews, *The Social World of Old Women: Management of Self-Identity*, Sage Publications, Inc., Beverly Hills, California, 1979.
25. G. C. Wenger, Personal Care: Variations in Network Type, Style, and Capacity, in *The Home Care Experience*, J. F. Gubrium and A. Sankar, (eds.), Sage Publications, Inc., Newbury Park, California, pp. 145-172, 1990.
26. C. L. Johnson and B. Barer, Families and Networks among Older Inner-City Blacks, *The Gerontologist, 30*, pp. 726-733, 1990.

# CHAPTER
7

# Bargaining for Care

*You got to give them something. They ain't gonna do something for you unless you do.*

Geraldine Starr

As much as she may hate it, Geraldine Starr knows that she must have help to meet her basic needs, and she knows that when people help her they incur costs. She believes that in order to get help from people she must offer something in return. Sometimes she fails in these attempts, getting neither what she wants nor what she needs.

Dowd views the dependence of older persons as the result of an unbalanced exchange relationship, in which others, because of the possession of greater resources, are in a position of power relative to more dependent persons [1]. Social interactions are seen as primarily an exchange of resources, and patterns of exchange are maintained over time because the people involved find the behavior rewarding. Although potentially rewarding, exchange behavior always entails costs, and the benefit derived from social exchange can be viewed as the difference between rewards and costs. Exchange behavior thus tends to continue as long as the behavior is perceived as more rewarding than costly.

When one exchange partner values the rewards more than the other, the relationship becomes unbalanced, and, from an exchange perspective, power is derived from the resulting imbalance. The dependence of one partner on another varies directly with the value of comparative resources and inversely with the availability of alternative exchange relationships [2]. Resources are essentially anything perceived as rewarding and include money, knowledge, persuasiveness, and social position [1].

The norm of reciprocity governs exchange relationships, and several kinds of reciprocity have been described [3]. Balanced reciprocity refers to exchanges where things of equal value are exchanged within a finite period of time and can be of two types—immediate and delayed. Immediate balanced reciprocity is appropriate when individuals wish to keep their obligation to a minimum, and such exchanges are instrumental and usually impersonal, for example, money. With delayed balanced reciprocity, gifts are offered with no stipulation for time of repayment, but since the receiver remains obligated to pay, an element of trust is introduced. Generalized reciprocity is the norm among close kin. In these relationships, the goods or services exchanged are not necessarily expected to be returned in exact proportion, if at all, and the assumption is that relationships will balance themselves out over the long term [4].

Much of the data related to informal support of elderly persons describes the caregiving relationship as one of reciprocal exchange. In spousal relationships, reciprocity is fairly balanced during the part of life when both spouses are relatively active, but when one spouse is severely impaired and requires comprehensive and continuing care, relationships are distinctly unbalanced. Caregiving then becomes quite stressful, and its continuation often depends on a long-standing, close relationship and is guided by the norm of generalized reciprocity [5-8].

The flow of support between parents and children also is frequently not one-way, but rather mutual, with parents continuing to furnish significant support to their adult offspring [4, 9-18]. As with husband-wife relations, data indicate that such support is based on a history of reciprocity [4, 19]. While the resources exchanged may not be equal, parents do offer both intrinsic and extrinsic rewards that children perceive as valuable.

The literature clearly affirms the presence of mutual support activity between generations in African American families [10, 12, 15, 20-24]. A number of studies suggest that this support is more important among blacks than whites [21, 23, 25, 26]. Other authors contend, however, that most differences can be attributed to socioeconomic status rather than to race [24, 27].

Among non-kin, research suggests that relationships also are generally reciprocal in nature. Data from several settings of age-segregated housing [14], an age-integrated inner-city neighborhood [9, 21], and a large national survey [10] indicate that the majority of residents participate in both instrumental and emotional exchanges, such as shopping, visiting, and helping out in sickness. In some cases, services were provided for a small fee, and exchanges were relatively balanced and involved little obligation; in other instances, exchanges were less equivalent, implying greater obligation [4, 28-35]. Occasionally, relationships resembled those between spouses or children in degree of attachment and level of care [4, 8, 30, 34]. Usually emotional attachment was present, and the rewards received in exchange for assistance included positive affect, gratitude, and small tokens.

Despite the typically reciprocal nature of informal caregiving relationships, numerous studies have confirmed the stress experienced by caregivers of frail elderly persons. Stress usually occurs because informal networks tend to respond to greater need by increasing the scope of assistance provided rather than by expanding in size [36]. Spouses who live with the elderly person are reported to suffer the most severe impact on everyday life [5]. Data show that children also endure a great deal of physical and emotional stress in providing care for functionally impaired parents [5, 6, 37-40]. Women are more subject to stress than men, since they have traditionally provided the most care and tended to reduce their leisure time rather than caregiving responsibilities in response to competing demands of marriage, children, and employment [5, 38, 40-42]. Non-kin typically incur fewer costs, primarily due to the fact that as a rule they are not the only persons providing care, and, of greater significance, non-kin generally do not assume comprehensive care of the more severely impaired or feel obligation to remain in relationships where imbalance is extreme [5, 7, 29, 43].

The literature suggests the utility of exchange theory as a theoretical tool to examine the informal caregiving relationships of these disabled old people. In this discussion we focus on the strategies they use to get help and on the costs of both giving and receiving care. We see that in situations where individuals have satisfactory, continuing relationships of exchange, relationships are for the most part relatively balanced and/or are governed by generalized reciprocity. Rev. Scott's relationship with Deacon Pate and Mrs. Finch's with her neighbor Doright are examples of balanced relationships, with sufficient rewards and few costs. The care of Mr. Oliver and Mr. Jones for their spouses exemplifies generalized reciprocity, where obligations incumbent in relationships are bound by strong kinship ties and a history of mutual help.

We also see that even in these situations of generalized reciprocity—when relationships are long-term and considerably unbalanced—significant stresses do occur. Mr. Oliver sometimes is overcome by the confinement of caregiving. In other cases, the burden of care is overwhelming because the caregiver has competing obligations or health problems or because the dependent person resists the care itself or the way in which it is offered.

In the previous chapter we saw that being the recipient of care also can be quite punishing. The stress of dependency derives from the loss of control that accompanies declining abilities, but it comes also from the feelings and emotions incumbent on being in the dependent role. Each of these participants has actively developed strategies aimed at getting needed help while at the same time trying to mitigate the costs of having it provided. These strategies involve various ways of increasing networks of support and interjecting obligation and trust into relationships. When possible, requests for help are accompanied by offers, both implicit and explicit, of rewards. It is clear here, and in the literature, that dependency is better accommodated by both parties when the care receiver can offer something in exchange for a service. Having valued resources to offer as rewards makes a difference, both in whether instrumental and affective needs are met and in the emotional impact of the caregiving experience.

Some of these informants manage to find helpers who do value the rewards exchanged for their caregiving activities, but often the resources they have to offer are not adequate to maintain a sufficient number of balanced relationships to meet their needs. Money, the resource most generally used to secure help by those individuals without relationships bound by strong kinship ties, is in short supply. Other resources tendered are typically minimal or simply not valued by caregivers. In some cases, either current or expected gains for caregivers are too scarce or the costs too high, and the dependent person achieves little success in bargaining for care. Those who can bear no longer the imbalance of a relationship often chose to abandon the quest for assistance and do without a needed service.

Our data make it clear that more is involved in the care situation than simply having a need for care and a person to perform a service, more than having resources to avoid dependency, to get rewards, or to reduce costs. It is also what goes on in the social interactions that are a necessary part of the caregiving process and the emotional effects of these interactions on the participants—how Mrs. Little feels when Mr. Avant "talks hateful" and how he feels when Mrs. Little complains about his cooking efforts. Also involved are the feelings associated with being burdensome and what it means when someone offers help freely or hesitates too long when responding to a request. These emotional costs must be a significant part of the cost-benefit analysis of the informal caregiving situation.

## OFFERING REWARDS

Each of these informants offers rewards for the care they receive. The type of rewards and the conditions under which they are extended determine the nature and the success of exchange relationships.

### Money

Even though money is scarce, it is commonly offered to informal caregivers. Some of these payments represent substantial portions of poverty-level incomes. Rev. Scott, pays Deacon Pate $40 a month for transportation and the variety of other services he regularly provides. Mrs. Finch gives her sister-in-law $25 to do her monthly shopping and to cash her checks. In other cases, more nominal fees are paid when the service is rendered, though these payments are usually for less significant services. Mrs. Little pays Rosa Mae $2 to go and get her beer or to help her get dressed, and Mrs. Finch gives Doright $1 every time he goes to the vegetable truck. Such cash remunerations have been noted in other studies of informal helping between impaired elders and non-kin caregivers [4, 28, 29].

Those who employ the strategy of paying informal helpers believe payment is necessary for the transaction to occur—both from the standpoint of the person performing the service and from that of the person requiring help. Geraldine Starr expresses the viewpoint that people expect more than gratitude for their services:

> Everybody's looking for something. They don't want no thanks. They say they can't spend it; they can't eat it.

Sally Finch agrees a cash payment is necessary, and, when one is dependent, also worth it:

> People don't bother with you unless you have money. I'm gonna give the money 'cause it's worth it. I can't get out and do for myself. Every time someone do something for you, you have to pay. Lots of people think he's [Doright] *got* to do, but he ain't, that he's supposed to do this for them, but he's not supposed to. They don't want to give him nothing for going. He don't go if they don't give him something. It's *worth* something when you can't do for yourself. Should give him a little something.

Rev. Scott believes that a dependent person has a moral obligation to pay for services, particularly when the services are significant, as Deacon Pate's have been:

Time I had nosebleed, I had to go to emergency clinic. He took me down there three times. Took me down there at ten o'clock at night, and it was daybreak when we came back. That was before he was taking any money. I just wouldn't listen [to his not taking the money]. I pay a cab—I feel like I can give him something.

For these persons needing help, offering the payment helps balance the relationship, making dependency more acceptable. The exchange relationships we observed resemble those found in other descriptions of reciprocal exchanges where reciprocity was usually of the immediate type when it appeared that the elderly person wanted to maintain a degree of independence or social distance. When real or perceived future needs existed, strategies were changed in an attempt to bring obligation and trust into the relationship [4].

Those transactions involving monthly fees, like those paid by Mrs. Finch and Rev. Scott, are delayed transactions and are calculated to instill greater obligation, offering more security to the dependent person with few alternatives for assistance. Mrs. Finch's only alternative for grocery shopping is her sister-in-law, and Rev. Scott must depend on Deacon Pate and his car to provide transportation for his many appointments since the public transportation service is too physically taxing. The security of a relationship—being able to count on a helper—is key. As Rev. Scott explains, the payment, particularly in transactions involving a monthly fee, can serve to formalize the relationship and engender stability:

I give him a small check each month because I have to have someone I can call on when I need him. Sometimes you ask people to do things for you once, and they won't take any money. Call them the second time, and you find they too busy to do something for you. They don't want to be bothered anymore.

Being poor often means that one's friends and family members also are poor, and this situation can create an advantageous position of exchange for the dependent person, keeping the relationships more balanced. Because Rosa Mae also depends on an income of only $386 per month, it is more likely she will find a ride to the liquor store to buy Mrs. Little's beer for the nominal payment of $2, an exchange that affords her the extra money she needs to buy cigarettes. In her ethnography of another poor black urban community, Stack discovered that situations of economic marginality fostered reciprocal exchanges [15]. Cantor and co-workers similarly suggested that the high degree of mutual aid present among black elderly women and their children living in New York City was related to their struggle for survival in a northern ghetto [9]. This situation of living on the financial edge means also that one offers payment when traditionally one might not—that is, with family members as well as with non-kin helpers. A common observation was that even families "charged."

On the other hand, poverty limits the amount of money these old people can pay for extra help, and when needs are extensive and prolonged, as in the case of Eloise Little, this strategy often is not a viable option. When Mrs. Little tried to pay market wages for help several hours a day, she soon had to abandon her plan:

> Gertrude sent that thirty-dollar [a day] woman here. I can't pay that thirty dollars a day. I don't have that kind of money. I had to quit 'cause I had to pay the water bill.

Caregivers do not always share the dependent person's perspective, and at times, the belief that one should pay friends and family members interferes with helping relationships. In the case of Geraldine Starr, it sometimes prevented her from accepting help from her husband's cousin, Ethel, who by Mrs. Starr's account often refused payment. Mrs. Starr's ideology supported the payment—that is, the payment was necessary and proper to continue the exchange relationship, especially since Ethel was not "blood kin." She also felt that she could not afford to pay what seemed to her an appropriate amount, now that Ethel, recently widowed, was in a less advantageous financial position:

> It don't make sense for her not to accept something when I offer. Sometime she do, and sometime she don't. It just hurts my heart, because she's so good, fill my freezer. I'm surprised she's so good to me for us to have no connection [blood relation]. I tell her to stop bringing stuff, but she keeps bringing it. If I don't give her money then I can't ask for nothing else. She got me sitting in a hole and I can't get out. I tried to give her $25, but she wouldn't accept it. When her husband was living she didn't have to worry about no bills. I told her I just wasn't able to give her $50. I wanted to give her $50 to pay for some of the things she brought me. I just wanted to give her some money. It was right for me to do. [But] I don't have no money worth nothing.

Paying Ethel was consistent with Mrs. Starr's belief that people's motivations are generally not altruistic and made her feel less obligated. Ethel's beliefs, however, differed, and because of these conflicts, at times Ethel stayed away for weeks. Wentowsky noted also that being able to offer even a small token in exchange bestowed feelings of independence, and when payment was refused, the service was considered an act of charity, making the recipient more reluctant to accept future help [4]. Fischer and colleagues similarly identified older persons who demonstrated their independence by insisting on paying nonfamily caregivers for services [29].

Not all informants believe that money is required, or even acceptable, and when beliefs do not support it, this strategy is not used. While Ms. Worth insists on offering money for gas, she does not pay her adopted children for their help because she has found offering money to be an ineffective strategy:

> It take gas to run cars. I offer it to you whether you accept it. Leonard doesn't accept 'less he see where he need it. They don't charge me though. But I appreciate it, and if I got anything, I'll offer any of you, if it's just gas. If I got anybody else, it would cost me more. You see what I'm saying? The way I look at it, you have somebody to help you and you don't have no money to be paying folks, 'cause you pay them sometimes and they don't do as good as they do voluntarily. I don't have nothing to offer but my kindness or something like that, my love.

## Other Rewards—In-Kind, Past, and Future

In cases of close socio-emotional bonds of kinship or friendship, rewards often have been tendered in the past, as in the situations of Lucy Oliver and Ruby Washington, whose husbands provide extensive care. Mr. Jones feels an obligation to care for his wife as she did for him during a period of disability following his job-related injury. These close kin relationships adhere to the principle of generalized reciprocity. This norm also governs the help Miss Fannie gives to Eloise Little—in this case based on her long-term relationship with Mrs. Little's now-deceased sister—and Rev. Scott's support from his niece, whom he helped send to college.

Although the literature is replete with evidence of children caring for the parents who once cared for them, we have seen that two of these older parents, Mrs. Starr and Ms. Worth, have little or no contact with living children. In both cases the child or children were not raised by their mothers, and no basis exists now for reciprocity.

Viola Worth has attempted to remedy this situation by adopting other kin—an active strategy sometimes used by older persons to obtain support when blood relationships are absent or unsatisfactory

[4, 26, 44, 45]. Ms. Worth, whose informal caregiving network is composed primarily of her adoptive children, has found this to be a useful strategy throughout her life:

> Just since I've growed up, I been claiming somebody for my children, I reckon since I've never had none. It's just nice to have somebody because families don't get along as well as I do here by myself. So many people got families. My family don't see after me the way my homemade family, my God-family, sees after me. I got one little nappy-headed son. He don't do nothing for me. I can't deny him because I brought him here [gave birth to him]. They hasn't done anything for me since I've been down. They wasn't fooling with me no way.

Because her blood son has not fulfilled the role of son as she defines it, she no longer views him in that role. Instead, she refers to her play children as her sons and daughters, and they call her, "Mama." Those with more primary roles in her care, Maxine and her mother, she has designated her "main" family and her god-family and has made it known to them that they are the ones she recognizes in her will, not her true son or his children. She even planned her own obituary—naming her play children first in her list of survivors.

While Ms. Worth has no money to bequeath, she does have a house, a significant potential reward for her goddaughter, Maxine, who is frequently unable to pay her rent. Barker and Mitteness described a similar situation—an elderly man who willed his house to his nonkin caregiver rather than to his own daughter [28]. Of course the value of a reward depends on how it is viewed by the prospective recipient. Mrs. Washington's house is a valuable resource because it provides her son and husband with needed shelter now and offers them a long-range reward after she is gone. Rev. Scott's brother and niece already have their own, more desirable, houses and because his other assets are minimal, he has little of value to offer as future rewards to his helpers.

Eloise Little's house has been a valuable resource in the past. When her roomer, Mr. Avant, first moved in with her, he provided daily care in return for a place to stay. When Mrs. Little's family started charging him rent, however, he stopped providing significant help, the costs for him outweighing the benefits:

> I used to sweep the porch everyday when I first moved here. Kept the house clean all the time, both refrigerators; cooked four times a day. Eloise Little was lookin' good. When they started charging me, I started doing less.

Neither can Mrs. Little offer her house as a future reward, since she shares ownership with her half-siblings, who will receive it no matter what they do or do not contribute to her care. She does offer temporary shelter from time to time to Eugene, her homeless and alcoholic nephew, a resource he values, but Mrs. Little receives almost nothing in return since Eugene himself has little of value to exchange:

> All he do is eat and walk the streets. I feed him and I give him a place to stay.

Interpersonal skills, what Weinstein terms "interpersonal competence," also can be valuable resources and are used regularly by some of these informants as less tangible rewards [46]. Viola Worth, as mentioned earlier, often has only her "kindness and love" to give, and she is careful to nurture relationships with her play children and her other helpers with these offerings. She is always mindful of the difficulties encountered by her caregivers, is considerate of their time, does not expect more than they can give, and shows her gratitude—all of which constitute valued rewards:

> I tell 'em, "Don't give me nothing," 'cause they give to me all the time. You know you appreciate things, but you don't be sittin' out there with no hand. You appreciate it. I tell all ya'll that. I appreciate what you do. There some people in the world that don't look at the good side, don't appreciate the little things what people do for them. I be grateful for little things. Some people find little things to grumble about. Matter of fact I appreciate everything. I appreciate from the little to the big. I appreciate little bitty things, and in my mind and my heart, that's when the big things will maybe come. It's nice to be thought of. That's the main thing. Some people easy to be forgotten, some ungrateful. They're gonna learn before they leave this world. That's why a lot of us don't get nowhere out there, because we always want the world and then don't appreciate it. We got to crawl before we can walk.

Ms. Worth's interpersonal competence has served her well over the years. She frequently states that she has always remembered the "golden rule," and she now reaps the bounty of her investment:

> It's the way you carry yourself. I try to treat you how I wish to be treated. All right, you good to me, I'll be good, kind or something, and if you see if there's anything you can do and you don't mind doing it. . . . You know, I think that sometime when a person get down, they were pretty cruel when they was up. You know you can't live in this world by yourself. You have to have somebody. I tell all

of ya'll I'm no saint, but I get my way, and I've tried to do the best I can. Now, I've had my ups and downs, and anybody, if they a human being, they gonna get angry sometimes, but I have treated people best I could. I've had my bitters and my sweets, but down through the years, I've treated people where people don't mind doing for me. See, that's what I'm saying. A lot of people when they get down, they don't have people come around because of the way they are. That's the way I look at it. That's the way it is with some people, they can be so stingy when they oughtn'. They ain't thinking about that time.

Lustbader noted similar benefits gained from having a history of reciprocity with potential helpers [47].

Mrs. Little, on the other hand, does not have Ms. Worth's generous nature, nor her interpersonal skills. According to Miss Fannie, who at one time provided daily care, she never has:

Eloise is a selfish person, never once thanked us, no gratitude. You got to be careful when you're going along. You don't know what you might need. She talks about Mr. Avant, "That old man burnt this and that," talk about anybody to you, talk about you, talked about him like he wasn't even in the house. Can't treat people like that if you can't do for yourself. I told Eloise that was all the family she had, and if she ran them off she wouldn't have anyone.

Neither has she ever tried to develop relationships, in this case with her half-sisters:

When Eloise was on her feet, she didn't associate with them. She didn't even claim them. She told Gertrude to her face, "You ain't none of my sister." She hurt her ownself. You got to be careful when you're going along. You don't know what you might need.

Other informants with limited informal support, such as Mrs. Finch and Mrs. Starr, also exhibit a less generous nature. Mrs. Finch confessed hiding a cake when her niece visited and expressed resentment that a sporadic helper, James, ate her food when she already had given him money. With Mrs. Starr, this tendency to avoid more costly reciprocal relationships is reinforced by her resistance to dependency:

I got my own troubles. I can't think about somebody else's troubles. She got a house note, the car. I just ain't got time to worry about the other person. I'm used to standing on myself. I can't get used to it. Got to learn to vouch for yourself.

Each of these women prefers to offer money for specific, time-limited services—with the goal of keeping their exchanges as balanced as possible and in the realm of business, rather than personal, transactions. Such behaviors coincide with historical attitudes negating the value of interdependent relationships. In contrast, cultivating relationships has been a critical element of Ms. Worth's lifelong creed:

> All my life I been trying to get along with people. Like that lady I was telling you about—just the way we met, I reckon. We just only met at, I don't know, out here at church or what, but I thank God. I don't know what it is. It's something about me—I meet certain people, we just stick together. It's just like you and I. You know what I mean? We didn't know one another, and now I'm crazy about you.

Her behavior is consistent with her personality and with her lifetime experience with disability.

## Last Resorts: Manipulation, Begging, and Compliance

When resources are scarce and no valued rewards can be offered, these dependent elders sometimes must resort to less acceptable strategies for getting help. Mrs. Oliver sometimes manipulates her children to make an unplanned visit by staging a health crisis on weekends. Matthews found this strategy to be common among old women in similarly disadvantageous positions vis-a-vis their children [48].

A more desperate last resort strategy is begging. Mrs. Little, with great need, few alternatives for care, and few valued resources, often is reduced to begging for needed help. When she telephones her sister-in-law to drive across town to rub her shoulders or when she asks Miss Fannie to come from next door to bring her a glass of water, her only resource—and one that frequently fails her—is the persuasiveness with which she can beg:

> I have to beg now. I don't have anybody to do anything for me. I just have to take what I can get.

Although Mrs. Little now often must resort to begging, Ms. Worth, with greater resources, is in a position to avoid this repugnant strategy:

> I may be a shut-in, but I don't beg.

Dowd noted that because of declining resources the aged often are forced to use compliance and respect as their exchange resources of last resort [1]. Although these informants, in their struggle to retain control, strive to avoid compliance, for people like Mrs. Little, sometimes little choice remains. Mrs. Little resisted for several years giving up the double bed she bought for herself when she was working, an accomplishment that gave her great pride, but she finally succumbed to her family's wishes and traded it for a hospital bed. Now, she often just listens in silence while they offer instructions about how she should manage her life. Miss Fannie commented recently on Mrs. Little's transformation:

> She was more humble. She wasn't runnin' nobody down. I felt sorry for her.

Because of this new humility, Miss Fannie has more compassion and a greater willingness to help.

## THE COSTS OF CAREGIVING

Even when these dependent elders have close ties of kinship, friendship, or valued resources to exchange with their caregivers, substantial stress is sometimes placed on family members and friends. At times these costs of caregiving are associated with the caregiver, other times with the persons needing care or their environment; often they are a combination of both.

Health problems frequently impede the role of caregivers [5, 7, 49] and are a factor in most of these caregiving situations. Mrs. Little's neighbor, Miss Fannie, at one time was a primary caregiver, providing extensive daily care, but she no longer is able assume this committed role due to her own heart trouble. Alcoholism interferes with Mrs. Little's nephew's ability to help, as well as with the quality of care provided to Mrs. Washington by her husband and son. In addition to hindering the caregiver's ability to help, health problems sometimes cause the dependent person to resist asking for or accepting help, as happened in the case of Mrs. Starr and her cousin, Ethel, who has severe rheumatoid arthritis:

> She upsets me very much. She don't set down. Have to stand up to cook. She swears she ain't hurtin', but she is hurtin'. She turns dark. I don't want her coming here and fallin' out. She ain't able to do anymore than I am. I didn't even call her.

Mrs. Finch avoids asking Doright to go with her to County because of his own advanced age and health problems:

> He ain't able, because he's too old. He might fall out on me. Look like he be as weak as I am.

On the other hand, older caregivers generally have more free time. Rev. Scott's helper, Deacon Pate, is happy to accept less than market wages for his services in exchange for an opportunity to perform a useful role that does not interfere unduly with his other activities:

> So as things are, I found Deacon Pate who had just retired and didn't have too much to do, and he didn't mind being helpful. He have time to take me places.

Where informal caregivers are younger, however, family and work responsibilities impose significant impediments to caring for these informants, even when ample affection and indebtedness are present. All of Ms. Worth's play children work, and Rev. Scott's niece has other obligations to her husband, child, and mother in a nursing home and to her full-time teaching job. Mrs. Finch's nephew has taken her sister—his other aunt who raised him—into his home, and her niece cares for two grandchildren while their mother is in the army overseas. Such competing obligations also interfere with assistance from Mrs. Oliver's children and Mrs. Little's half-sister, Gertrude.

Sometimes the barriers to care stem from certain objectionable traits in the dependent person. Eloise Little, in addition to having many needs and being resource-poor, is extremely difficult to please. Miss Fannie, who used to cook for her daily, explains the frustration of trying to help someone who rarely is satisfied with her efforts:

> I've tried everything. Eloise just don't like food. She's real peculiar in her own way. She is very particular about her food. You can't get it right. You have to wash grits and rice and oatmeal three times, get every little speck out. I never could buy beef to suit her—brisket too fat, boneless beef too dry. You can't please her. She's a mess. I went over there everyday, even when ice on the ground. I would put it in a little tub with cover so it wouldn't spill. I tried to fix food the way she liked.

Mr. Avant, the recipient of similar abuse from Mrs. Little, emphasizes the off-putting impact of such behavior:

> Eloise can be so mean. That's what made me so mad when I was cooking for her—mess over good food, send it back four or five times. She's going to have to change her eating habits—stop asking people to fix things she isn't going to eat.

In her own occasional role as caregiver, the first author experienced similar maltreatment by Geraldine Starr, who also is difficult to satisfy and regularly complains about services rendered or items purchased. At times she loses her temper, lashing out at the person trying to help. She admits to having difficult ways:

> Yeah, I'm fitified, got some funny ways. I been crabbish all my life. I try to put the brakes on it. I'm grown. I don't have to lie about it.

Others have noted similar ill-natured responses, as well as complete resistance of caregiving efforts [47, 50]. In his study of nursing home life, Savishinsky described helpless residents who lashed out in anger at those trying to care for them [50]. He surmised that each attempt to help only made residents feel even more helpless, reminding them of their own dependence.

Viola Worth, on the other hand, is shrewd enough to recognize the potential harm of such behavior and employs a more fertile strategy:

> It's hard to shop for anyone. I'm trying to let you know I'm not choicy. Just do the best you can.

The costs of caregiving can be either minimized or magnified by the actions of the care receiver. As noted, Ms. Worth always offers her kindness and consideration in exchange for the time her caregivers devote to her despite their busy schedules. She also realizes that by trying to help herself, she can further reduce her own costs and those of her caregivers as well:

> There are some even in my business that they don't want to try to help theirselves. You know it makes it hard on folks. Look, you try to help me. You ain't *got* to, ain't nobody got to do nothing. Everybody know Viola trying to help herself.

Sometimes the symptoms that accompany illness, in addition to preventing self-care, can make caregiving still more demanding. The depression and anxiety that deter Mrs. Starr's and Mrs. Finch's ability to function also appear to hinder the inclination of others to help. For when inquiries are made of Mrs. Starr about her condition, her replies are nearly always embittered, usually including a litany of her many ailments, and her low moods rarely are improved by her caregivers' efforts. And Sally Finch's acrimonious actions toward her niece's children, heightened by her nervous condition, discourage all but occasional visits:

> Them's [the children] the baddest things. Don't want to be bothered
> with children. They pull down everything. She [her niece] won't
> hardly touch 'em. They're gonna make her cry one day. Me and my
> sister talk about it. You're supposed to teach a child. She don't want
> you to spank them. That's why she don't come around. I try to tell
> her. She'll learn one day. She lets them have their way, do just
> what they want to. I be done broke their necks. She just talks to
> them.

Clearly, Mrs. Finch's attitudes toward childrearing, being incompatible
with those of her niece, create additional strain and prevent counting
such advice among valued rewards she can offer.

The pain experienced by the dependent person also can increase the
burden of caregiving. Eloise Little's cries of pain while being changed
or rubbed magnifies the stress of performing such tasks. Mrs. Oliver's
speech impediments and cognitive impairments make visits with her
less enjoyable, and when individuals are wheelchair-bound, tasks that
involve taking them out clearly are more arduous and sometimes
impossible.

When the needs for care are extreme, the costs experienced during
the helping process can outweigh any benefits the dependent person
has to offer. Mrs. Little's half-sister, Marion, explains how the strain of
caregiving contributes to the sporadic nature of her assistance:

> Eloise works my eyeballs out when I come over there. I have to
> learn to wind down, try not to do everything. It's depressing coming
> over here. When it gets to me, I just have to stay away for a few
> weeks.

Conflicts between caregivers sometimes exacerbate already difficult
circumstances and increase the stress for all concerned. Instead of
rallying a cooperative effort to meet her heavy care needs, Mr. Avant
and Mrs. Little's half-sisters squabble amongst themselves, often voicing opinions about each other's inadequacies:

> Her sisters don't take good care of her. I wouldn't treat my sister
> that way. They fight with each other, talk about what the other
> does or doesn't do. Tom always complaining he doesn't have time to
> get the Chux [protective bed pads]. They always singing the blues.

## DOING WITHOUT

As we have seen, significant costs also can be incurred by the care
receiver. Sometimes the costs associated with being helped are so

troublesome the dependent person chooses to resist the help offered and do without a needed service.

Costs related to real or perceived attempts at control by caregivers are regularly avoided by care receivers. Even in her disadvantageous position, Mrs. Little resists control of her personal space and in so doing impedes her half-sisters' attempts, albeit infrequent, to help:

> We do what she lets us do. She keeps us at arm's length. We can't break her system. You know she won't let you touch anything. Hope we didn't throw away too much. We saved two or three of everything. She need to let somebody clean up that room. It's a fire hazard.

Mrs. Little routinely defies Mr. Avant's attempts to control her behavior, cutting off another avenue to needed help:

> Told me to drink milk everyday. I don't need no man telling me what to do. I don't ask him no more.

Because of her desire for independence as well as her need to retain control over how household tasks are done, Mrs. Starr curtails the efforts of her cousin Ethel:

> I told her, "Stay at home. Let me do a little something. Let me fall out myself." She wants to do things the way *she* wants to do. I tell her to stop bringing stuff, but she keeps bringing it. She turned the burners up too high. I told her not to. She didn't like that too much.

Feelings of being burdensome frequently prevent these elders from asking for and accepting help. Such feelings encourage Mrs. Starr's adamant refusal to call on her other cousin Dorothy when she has one of her frequent falls:

> I try not to bother Dorothy no more than I can help. I don't want to bother her period! I'll lay on this floor till day, just like I have laid. I don't want to bother nobody! I have been where I could get up. Now I can't get up. I'm not like that. I'm not going to fall on top of them.

As discussed in the previous chapter, the likelihood that help will be spurned is increased by a perceived reluctance on the part of the

caregiver. We see how Rev. Scott's understanding of his niece's competing loyalties, compounded by his perception of foot-dragging on her
part, leads him to refuse her offer to bring dinner:

> Last Saturday night I told her I had some food, so she didn't need to
> come. She have enough on her without me adding to her burden.
> Sometimes she sound like she don't have time.

Less subtle negative reactions, like those Mrs. Little sometimes
receives from Mr. Avant, almost ensure a care receiver's resolve
to do without:

> He talks to me so hateful. Call him to cut off the fan, he'll cut my
> throat. I don't call him no more. He always got something to say.
> Sometimes I do without water all day long. My feelings are easily
> hurt.

Lustbader noted that some impaired persons find it easier to "fold
into the necessity of getting help" [47, p. 9]. We also found that while
each of these seven elders values independence, some adapt better to
being helped. A number of factors may contribute to differences in
adaptability. Ms. Worth, who often claims a lifelong "affliction," accepts
more easily her need for help, still holding dear her ideal of independence. Her adaptability may be related to the continuity of her
handicapped identity, as Rubinstein and colleagues [51] suggested
about the elders they studied.

Wenger proposed a relationship between patterns of behavior in
earlier, healthier lives and later adaptations to dependency [52]. She
found old people in Wales who were accustomed to living with or
near relatives had built up patterns of behavior based on availability
and expectation of help, while those without close relatives developed
expectations of self-reliance that continued into old age. In our study,
the two women who lived with their spouses and also had children close
by, were less troubled by various aspects of being helped, especially
when that help was provided by these close family members.

Mrs. Worth does not place as much value on the equity of exchanges
and accepts more easily unbalanced relationships. Roberto noted that,
in friendships between older adults, an individual's personality could
influence the importance attached to equity between friends and that
those individuals without strong beliefs in equity were less uncomfortable occupying inferior exchange positions [53].

The impact of dependency radiates into all aspects of these
participants' lives. Stoller [16] reported lower morale among dependent

persons who had nothing to offer family caregivers in exchange for their help, and, as noted in Chapter 4, Rook [54] found that older women who were either overbenefited or underbenefited in their relationships with their informal supporters expressed greater feelings of loneliness than women in more balanced relationships. We have seen reduction in social interactions and loneliness and observed how some participants relate loss of friends to their impairments. Certainly, their needs, coupled with their inabilities often to reciprocate, have contributed to these situations.

* * * * *

The attitudes and behaviors relating to the informal component of long-term care embody the complexity that is evident in other aspects of the long-term care situation. The impact of this complexity on how some dependent persons view their caregiving needs is portrayed effectively in Geraldine Starr's plaintive and revealing outburst:

> I don't know what I want myself. Lord, what must I do? What's going to become of me? I don't want to suffer. I try to get up and do. I don't want to fall no more.

Here, Mrs. Starr expresses her despair at being chronically impaired and losing her independence, at being in a situation where, from her point of view, no acceptable solutions to her problems are possible. This definition of reality creates an ambivalence of attitudes and behaviors that imposes its own constraints on the caregiving process, that makes providing care to her a formidable task. Getting and receiving care are not problematic in quite the same way or to the same degree for all of these participants, but in each case both processes are complex, dynamic, and difficult.

By using the theoretical perspective of exchange to view the situation of dependency, we have related the problems of these individuals to their declining resources—resources both to practice self-care and to use as barter in exchange relationships, and we have evaluated their actions in terms of rewards and costs and attempts to balance caregiving relationships. These ways of viewing the informal caregiving situation clarify the meanings of behaviors and, in so doing, afford greater understanding of both the objective and the more subjective needs for formal services—needs of the caregiver as well as those of the dependent person.

It is clear that the value placed by these frail elders on preserving independence has a major impact on their informal caregiving relationships. This value influences the strategies they use to take care of their own needs rather than asking for or accepting help; it influences their decisions to remain in their own homes rather than move in with family members; it influences their selection of social interactions; it influences the ways they present themselves to their caregivers; and it influences the strategies they use to get help and reduce the costs of being helped. In Part III we address the formal caregiving system—first describing the impact of formal services on the lives of these individuals and then examining various aspects of the formal care relationship. We see that some of the same beliefs and values guide the actions and reactions of these informants in their associations with their formal caregivers. The primacy of the value for independence is unmistakable.

## REFERENCES

1. J. Dowd, Aging as Exchange: A Preface to Theory, *Journal of Gerontology, 30,* pp. 584-594, 1975.
2. J. Dowd, Exchange Rates and Old People, *Journal of Gerontology, 35,* pp. 596-602, 1980.
3. M. Sahlins, On the Sociology of Primitive Exchange, in *The Relevance of Models for Social Anthropology,* M. Banton (ed.), Praeger, New York, 1965.
4. G. J. Wentowski, Reciprocity and the Coping Strategies of Older People: Cultural Dimensions of Network Building, *The Gerontologist, 21,* pp. 600-609, 1981.
5. M. Cantor, Strain among Caregivers: A Study of Experience in the United States, *The Gerontologist, 23,* pp. 597-604, 1983.
6. C. L. Johnson, Dyadic Family Relations and Social Support, *The Gerontologist, 23,* pp. 377-383, 1983.
7. C. L. Johnson and D. J. Catalano, Childless Elderly and their Family Supports, *The Gerontologist, 21,* pp. 610-618, 1981.
8. K. Jonas and E. Wellin, Dependency and Reciprocity: Home Health Aid in an Elderly Population, in *Aging in Culture and Society: Comparative Viewpoints and Strategies,* C. Fry (ed.), J. F. Bergin, Brooklyn, 1980.
9. M. Cantor, Life Space and the Social Support System of the Inner City Elderly of New York, *The Gerontologist, 15,* pp. 23-27, 1975.
10. L. R. Hatch, Informal Support Patterns of Older African-American and White Women, *Research on Aging, 13*:2, pp. 144-170, 1991.
11. H. Kendig and D. Rowland, Family Support of the Australian Aged: Comparison with the United States, *The Gerontologist, 23,* pp. 643-649, 1983.
12. J. Mitchell and J. C. Register, An Exploration of Family Interaction with the Elderly by Race, Socioeconomic Status and Residence, *The Gerontologist, 24,* pp. 48-54, 1984.

13. E. Shanas, The Family as a Social Support System in Old Age, *The Gerontologist, 19*, pp. 64-69, 1979.
14. S. Sherman, Mutual Assistance and Support in Retirement Housing, *Journal of Gerontology, 30*, pp. 479-483, 1975.
15. C. Stack, *All Our Kin*, Harper and Row, New York, 1974.
16. E. Stoller, Exchange Patterns in the Informal Networks of the Elderly: The Impact on Morale, *Journal of Marriage and the Family, 47*, pp. 851-857, 1985.
17. M. B. Sussman, The Family Life of Old People, in *Handbook of Aging and the Social Sciences*, R. H. Binstock and E. Shanas (eds.), Van Nostrand Reinhold, New York, pp. 218-243, 1976.
18. W. K. Vicusi, An Assessment of Aid to the Elderly: Incentive Effects and the Elderly's Role in Society, in *Aging, Stability, and Family Change*, J. March (ed.), Academic Press, New York, 1981.
19. A. James, W. L. James, and H. L. Smith, Reciprocity as a Coping Strategy of the Elderly: A Rural Irish Perspective, *The Gerontologist, 24*, pp. 483-489, 1984.
20. J. Aschenbrenner, *Lifelines: Black Families in Chicago*, Holt, Rinehart, and Winston, New York, 1975.
21. M. Cantor, Neighbors and Friends: An Overlooked Resource in Informal Support System, *Research on Aging, 1*:4, pp. 434-463, 1979.
22. R. C. Gibson and J. S. Jackson, The Health, Physical Functioning, and Informal Supports of the Black Elderly, *The Milbank Quarterly, 65*, pp. 421-454, 1987.
23. W. C. Hays and C. H. Mindel, Extended Kinship Relations in Black and White Families, *Journal of Marriage and the Family, 35*, pp. 51-57, 1973.
24. J. J. Jackson, *Minorities and Aging*, Wadsworth Publishing Co., Belmont, California, 1980.
25. A. C. Hill and F. Jaffe, Negro Fertility and Family Size Preferences: Implications for Programming of Health and Social Services, in *The Black Family: Essays and Studies*, R. Staples (ed.), Wadsworth Publishing Co., Belmont, California, 1971.
26. C. L. Johnson and B. Barer, Families and Networks Among Older Inner-City Blacks, *The Gerontologist, 30*, pp. 726-733, 1990.
27. E. Mutran, Intergenerational Family Support among Blacks and Whites: Response to Culture or to Socioeconomic Differences, *Journal of Gerontology, 40*:3, pp. 382-389, 1985.
28. J. C. Barker and L. S. Mitteness, Invisible Caregivers in the Spotlight: Non-kin Caregivers of Frail Older Adults, in *The Home Care Experience*, J. F. Gubrium and A. Sankar (eds.), Sage Publications, Inc., Newbury Park, California, 1990.
29. L. R. Fischer, L. Rogne, and N. N. Eustis, Support Systems for the Family-less Elderly: Care Without Commitment, in *The Home Care Experience*, J. F. Gubrium and A. Sankar (eds.), Sage Publications, Inc., Newbury Park, California, 1990.

30. C. C. Goodman, Natural Helping Among Older Adults, *The Gerontologist, 24*, pp. 138-143, 1984.
31. A. Hochschild, *The Unexpected Community*, Prentice Hall, Englewood Cliffs, New Jersey, 1973.
32. N. Rosel, The Hub of a Wheel: A Neighborhood Support Network, *International Journal of Aging and Human Development, 16*, pp. 193-200, 1983.
33. J. K. Ross, *Old People, New Lives: Community Creation in a Retirement Residence*, University of Chicago Press, Chicago, 1977.
34. J. Smithers, *Determined Survivors: Community Life Among the Urban Elderly*, Rutgers University Press, New Brunswick, New Jersey, 1985.
35. J. Sokolovsky and C. Cohen, Being Old in the Inner City: Support Systems of the SRO Aged, in *Aging in Culture and Society: Comparative Viewpoints and Strategies*, C. Fry (ed.), J. F. Bergin, Brooklyn, pp. 163-181, 1980.
36. E. P. Stoller and K. L. Pugliesi, Size and Effectiveness of Informal Helping Networks: A Panel Study of Older People in the Community, *Journal of Health and Social Behavior, 32*, pp. 180-191, 1991.
37. E. K. Abel, Daughters Caring for Elderly Parents, in *The Home Care Experience*, J. F. Gubrium and A. Sankar (eds.), Sage Publications, Inc., Newbury Park, California, 1990.
38. E. Brody, "Women in the Middle" and Family Help to Older People, *The Gerontologist, 21*, pp. 471-480, 1981.
39. B. Robinson and M. Thurhner, Taking Care of Aged Parents, *The Gerontologist, 19*, pp. 586-593, 1979.
40. E. Stoller, Parental Caregiving by Adult Children, *Journal of Marriage and the Family, 45*, pp. 851-858, 1983.
41. R. Stone, G. L. Cafferata, and J. Sangl, Caregivers of the Frail Elderly: A National Profile, *The Gerontologist, 27*:5, pp. 616-626, 1987.
42. J. Treas, Family Support Systems for the Aged, *The Gerontologist, 17*, pp. 486-491, 1977.
43. C. L. Johnson and D. J. Catalano, A Longitudinal Study of Family Supports to the Impaired Elderly, *The Gerontologist, 23*, pp. 612-618, 1983.
44. K. R. Allen and V. Chin-Sang, A Lifetime of Work: The Context and Meanings of Leisure for Aging Black Women, *The Gerontologist, 30*:6, pp. 734-740, 1990.
45. H. MacRae, Fictive Kin as a Component of the Social Networks of Older People, *Research on Aging, 14*:2, pp. 226-247, 1992.
46. E. Weinstein, The Development of Interpersonal Competence, in *Handbook of Socialization Theory and Research*, D. Goslin (ed.), Rand McNally, Chicago, 1969.
47. W. Lustbader, *Counting on Kindness: The Dilemmas of Dependency*, The Free Press, New York, 1991.
48. S. Matthews, *The Social World of Old Women: Management of Self-Identity*, Sage Publications, Inc., Beverly Hills, California, 1979.
49. J. McCann, Long-term Home Care for the Elderly: Perceptions of Nurses, Physicians, and Primary Caregivers, *QRB, 18*, pp. 66-74, 1988.

50. J. Savishinsky, *The Ends of Time: Life and Work in a Nursing Home*, Bergin and Garvey, New York, 1991.
51. G. C. Wenger, Personal Care: Variations in Network Type, Style, and Capacity, in *The Home Care Experience*, J. F. Gubrium and A. Sankar (eds.), Sage Publications, Inc., Newbury Park, California, pp. 145-172, 1990.
52. R. L. Rubinstein, J. C. Kilbride, and S. Nagy, *Elders Living Alone*, Aldine de Gruyter, New York, 1992.
53. K. A. Roberto, Equity in Friendships, in *Older Adult Friendships*, R. G. Adams and R. Blieszner (eds.), Sage Publications, Inc., Newbury Park, California, pp. 147-165, 1989.
54. K. S. Rook, Reciprocity of Social Exchange and Social Satisfaction Among Older Women, *Journal of Personality and Social Psychology, 62*, pp. 145-154, 1987.

# Part III
# The Formal Care Experience

# CHAPTER
# 8

# The Role of Formal Care

*I was trying to tell Gertrude that nobody comes on the weekend. She can't understand it. She say I need somebody everyday. I say I sure do. I need loving everyday and every night. I think I need somebody to come in and cook me one good meal. I'm laying here hungry from one day to another.*

Eloise Little

Once Mr. Avant slips past Eloise Little's bed on his early morning mission of unlocking her door, she routinely is left alone until one of her aides arrives. On Mondays and Thursdays, the days her homemaker aide is scheduled, this visit could be as early as 8:00 or 9:00 A.M. On the other weekdays Mrs. Little usually has to wait till at least early afternoon for a visit. She waits also, except on rare occasions when an informal helper drops by, for her first meal of the day and to have her clothes or diaper changed. On weekends, when no aides come, Mrs. Little is completely dependent on her informal caregiving network.

The goal of community-based care is to allow individuals to remain in their own home and enjoy a better quality of life. For some of these clients this goal is achieved with resounding success. For others the impact of the formal care component is slight. Eloise Little receives the maximum level of services allowed through Georgia's Community Care Services Program and her other providers. Yet, as her woeful words convey, her situation remains desperate.

The discussion thus far of these seven elders has portrayed a wide range of needs and informal caregiving arrangements—from Mrs. Little, bedridden, helpless, and often alone with no one even to bring her a glass of water, to Viola Worth, proud and happy to be able to do so many things for herself and bolstered by her "homemade family." But for each person, some basic needs for care remain—needs that cannot be met either by their own self-care activities or by their informal caregiving networks. Because of these unmet needs, each person receives additional services through the formal component of the caregiving system. Since these services are meant to supplement those provided by informal caregivers, the extent and types of formal services reflect the effectiveness of the informal care system and the abilities of the clients to maintain themselves.

We now turn our attention to the formal care experiences of the seven informants whose lives we are sharing. The focus will be on the care they receive in their homes from home care aides, often described as the "backbone" of home care [1]. Although each person receives other formal services, these paraprofessionals provide the bulk of their formal care. We begin with a description of the complex system of care that delivers formal services to these clients and a discussion of the impact these services have on each client's long-term care situation.

## THE FORMAL CAREGIVING SYSTEM

For each of these seven clients, the Community Care Services Program (CCSP) provides, or at one time was providing, the greater part of their community-based services. Each person has been enrolled in CCSP for at least three years; three have been receiving CCSP services for five years. CCSP provides for client assessment, case management, and for a range of other services, including:

- Adult Day Rehabilitation (ADR);
- Alternative Living Services (ALS), health-related support services in a residential setting (e.g., personal care or board and care home);
- Home-delivered health services, including home health aides (HHA), personal care aides (PCA), homemaker aides (HMA)*, respite care, nursing care, medical social work, speech therapy, and physical therapy; and
- Emergency Response System (ERS), an in-home electronic support system providing clients with a twenty-four-hour, seven-day-a-week access to a medical control center.

Organization and administration of CCSP is complex. Entry into the program requires a referral, which may come from a variety of sources, including physicians, hospitals, community organizations,

*CCSP now has combined personal care aide services and homemaker aide services into a new designation—personal support aide (PSA).

family members, and friends. Prospective clients must be Medicaid-eligible, or potentially Medicaid-eligible within 180 days and be certified by a physician for skilled or intermediate nursing home care. Clients are assessed for their functional and financial eligibility by a team made up of a registered nurse (RN) and a caseworker under the supervision of the County Health Department. Once eligibility is determined, the assessment team develops an initial plan for the client's care. Additional assessments are conducted on an annual basis and when a change in condition warrants.

Clients are referred to CCSP case managers, who use these assessments to plan and coordinate individual services. Case managers, who are employees of a private non-profit agency that oversees a number of programs for older persons, make regular home visits every three months to review client services. They are responsible for all the paperwork involved in communicating with the assessment team and the various agencies that deliver the services.

The services planned for each client are provided by a variety of for-profit home health care agencies and non-profit organizations. Each provider also has its own in-house coordinator for CCSP clients as well as an RN supervisor for each client. The RN supervisor visits the client regularly to oversee aide services and to determine whether or not skilled nursing is required. The case manager, as well as the supervisory RN from the home health agency, may specify services appropriate for each client. The designated services are contracted by CCSP from a number of different home health and service providers.

In addition to the services provided through CCSP (Medicaid-funded), all of these individuals receive home-delivered services furnished by other programs or organizations. Medicare typically pays for home-health services when health conditions become more acute, as after hospitalization, or when frequent skilled nursing care is required. In most cases, Medicare services are furnished by the same agencies that provide CCSP services; however, CCSP case managers are not involved in their management. Some clients have homemaker aides provided by either the County Department of Family and Children's Services (DFACS) or the local housing authority. Home-delivered meal service (Meals-on-Wheels) is provided by the same non-profit organization furnishing CCSP case management. Medicaid-funded medical transportation services are contracted out to various commercial health transport services, with oversight by service workers in the Department of Family and Children's Services. Additional transportation services are furnished to public housing tenants by the housing authority.

## THE FORMAL CARE PLAN

As the preceding description of the formal system illustrates, each client's care plan involves numerous organizations, often resulting in a complex and bewildering array of providers. For example, Eloise Little is assigned a CCSP case manager, two additional service managers from two separate home health care agencies, a coordinator at the Meals-on-Wheels office, a service worker at DFACS who handles transportation eligibility, and a transportation dispatcher, all of whom she must contact when she has problems or needs their services. A different line-up of individuals actually provide the services in her home—RN's and aides (who sometimes change) from two provider agencies; volunteers who deliver meals, a different one daily; and assessors, not always the same one, from the County Health Department. During the normal course of service delivery, Mrs. Little might have contact with as many as fifteen different individuals, each of whom is either providing or supervising her care. In a typical week she is visited by a minimum of seven formal workers, some of whom are not aware of the visits of the others or of their roles in Mrs. Little's care.

For each of these seven clients, services evolved as the individual's situation or needs changed. These changes involved either an increase or decrease in a particular service, a change in providers, or a switch from CCSP to Medicare. After her hip replacement, Medicare assumed coverage of Ms. Worth's services in order to provide more frequent monitoring and physical therapy. Similarly, Rev. Scott required skilled nurses to change his bandages after his skin graft. In these two cases, Medicare services were temporary, but when conditions warrant, Medicare coverage may be extended. Mrs. Washington, Mrs. Little, and Mrs. Oliver each received home-delivered services under Medicare for over a year. Because Mrs. Washington's condition was not expected to improve and she was receiving no other CCSP services, she was terminated, retaining only the Medicare home health services.

Geraldine Starr's CCSP services have been interrupted twice since she entered the program. The first time, a period of a year, was the result of a mix-up in providers, only clarified when her senior companion intervened. Mrs. Starr then was receiving home health aide services twice a week and weekly RN services from another home care provider, ordered after back surgery and continuing for a period of five months until a duplication of services was discovered. All CCSP services were suspended a second time for three months, when Mrs. Starr fell and broke her hip, requiring a subsequent hospitalization and nursing home stay. Her services resumed at their former level when she returned home.

Table 1 depicts the year of entry into CCSP and the services provided to each client at the end of the study period. Although our focus throughout the discussion of the formal care experience relates primarily to the services provided by home care aides, a better understanding of their services and of the "mosaic" [2] of each client's care will be afforded by knowing the complete array of formal services.

**TABLE 1**
Client Care Plans: Source, Frequency, Type of Services

| | Entry Date | CCSP | Medicare | DFACS | Public Housing | OAA Agency |
|---|---|---|---|---|---|---|
| Eloise Little | 1987 | HMA 2/wk RN 1/mo ERS | HHA 5/wk | TRANS* | | MOW |
| Ruby Washington | 1986 | | HHA 5/wk RN 2/mo | TRANS* | | MOW |
| Viola Worth | 1985 | PCA 3/wk RN Bi-mo | | TRANS* | | MOW |
| Joseph Scott | 1987 | PCA 4/wk HMA 1/wk RN 2/mo | | TRANS* | | |
| Lucy Oliver | 1987 | ADR 3/wk RESPITE 2/wk | HHA 2/wk RN 2/mo | TRANS* | | |
| Geraldine Starr | 1987 | HMA 5/wk RN 1/mo ERS | | TRANS* | TRANS** HMA 1/wk | |
| Sally Finch | 1985 | PCA 3/wk | HMA Bi-mo | | | |

HMA — Homemaker Aide
HHA — Home Health Aide
PCA — Personal Care Aide
RN — Registered Nurse
ERS — Emergency Response System
MOW — Meals on Wheels
OAA — Older Americans Act

*Transportation for medical purposes
**Transportation for non-medical purposes

## THE IMPACT OF AIDE SERVICES

As the client's care plans indicate, most formal care delivered in their homes is provided by home care aides. Four persons (Mrs. Little, Mrs. Starr, Mrs. Washington, and Rev. Scott) have services from some type of aide five days a week; three receive regular care from two different types of aides; Mrs. Little and Mrs. Starr sometimes have two aides (in 2 categories or from 2 organizations) present on the same day.

Aides are authorized to provide specific services. Personal care aides (PCA's) typically assist clients with bathing, dressing, and some household tasks associated with personal care. They may also help with medications if appropriate. Home health aides (HHA's) perform more skilled health care such as taking vital signs and flushing catheters. Homemaker aides (HMA's) overlap some components of the other two and are designed to help with personal care tasks as well as essential household activities, which may include housecleaning, shopping, laundry, and bill paying. The length of time personal care and homemaker aides are scheduled per visit ranges from one to two hours. Home health aides have no specified time allotted, but a typical visit lasts approximately forty-five minutes. The intended role of all of these aides is to fill in the gaps—to carry out those home care tasks that neither clients nor their informal caregivers are able to accomplish.

A great deal of variability exists in the kinds of services performed by aides and in the significance of their roles in each of these client's lives. Some of these differences can be attributed to the type of aide performing the service. As noted, agency regulations indicate the kind of care each type of aide may provide; in addition, each client has an individualized plan of care. We will see, however, that the real situation—the tasks that these aides actually perform—often deviates from the authorized program. We found, as have others [3, 4], that each type of aide frequently performs tasks in each category of home care (ADL, IADL, and health care), some aides go far beyond the functions specified for them in the guidelines, and other aides fall short of the expected role.

Our data show the typical role of home health aide involves, as the guidelines specify, tasks related to health care and personal care, such as taking vital signs and helping with bathing, hair care, dressing, medication, and mobility. Only on occasion do home health aides provide nutrition-related services, such as picking up fast-food or, more rarely, cooking a meal, but such events are exceptions. Except for Mrs. Washington's aide, who regularly sweeps the floor in the room where

Mrs. Washington stays, the only IADL task typically performed by home health aides is changing bed linens. In no situation is the home health aide involved in management of care.

The role of personal care aides varies widely among the three individuals who receive services. Ms. Worth's PCA performs a range of tasks on a regular basis, including all three areas of care—ADL, IADL, and health care. She often assumes a managerial role, reminding Ms. Worth about her medicine and keeping up with her medical appointments. She has become involved with her client on a more personal level as well—bringing her gifts on special occasions and dinner on Christmas day. Mrs. Finch's personal care aide, however, regularly only does routine personal care chores, and the aide that helps Rev. Scott has a similar function, with the addition of minimal cooking.

Homemaker aides typically perform a wider variety of services, including both personal care and housekeeping tasks, as well as some health care assistance. In each situation, however, the role of the homemaker aide varies. Rev. Scott's homemaker aide assumes the bulk of his housekeeping, shopping, and cooking chores on a regular basis, but she provides no personal care or health care, except as it relates to nutrition. In Mrs. Little's case, the homemaker aide does mostly personal care and a minimal amount of IADL and health care chores. Mrs. Starr's homemaker performs some tasks in all three areas but does none on a regular basis.

Even with the care supplied by these aides, by other formal caregivers, and by family and friends, some of these impaired elders still have unmet needs for care—some quite significant. Mrs. Little has many residual needs, including basic daily care. If she has a bowel movement after the aide has left or on weekends, she has to lie in her own filth for hours or even days if she cannot find a neighbor or visitor to help. Her formal care services have failed to produce significant impact on the unkept state of her house. Mice and roaches thrive amid the containers of uneaten meals scattered around on her bed and tables; the refrigerator is full of rotting food; and soiled bed linens and gowns typically are found in the broken washing machine in the kitchen. Her prescribed medicine is rarely taken, medical appointments sometimes slip by unnoted, and clinic visits are usually unaccompanied. She is frequently lonely and hungry.

While other individuals also have deficiencies in home care, none are as critical as Mrs. Little's. Mrs. Starr's expressed needs primarily revolve around food shopping and preparation, but when her symptoms are more severe, she needs help with other housekeeping chores and with her medications. Mrs. Finch has unmet health care needs—

getting to the hospital, getting around the hospital, and obtaining her medicine. Although in the past her aide was able to go with her, program restrictions no longer permit this service.

Even with extensive informal help from primary caregivers, the supplemental formal assistance still leaves Mrs. Washington and Mrs. Oliver with unmet needs. Mrs. Washington's house is often dirty, and she has no transportation for non-medical purposes. Mrs. Oliver sometimes does not take her medicine correctly or eat appropriately for her diabetic condition, and her husband frequently expresses a need for additional respite from his caregiving role.

The following passages depict the impact of the care from aides.

## ELOISE LITTLE

Eloise Little receives home health aide services and homemaker aide services from two different agencies. After a change in HHA's about three months into the study, Mrs. Little has kept the same two aides—Annette and Janice.

Annette, the home health aide, is scheduled to come Monday through Friday; her visits last from thirty minutes to two hours, but typically do not exceed an hour. When Mrs. Little was still able to get out of her bed to use the portable commode, Annette's usual chores were to empty the commode and the trash and take Mrs. Little's vital signs. Now that Mrs. Little is bed-bound and has to wear diapers and use a urinary catheter, Annette also cleans her and her bed after bowel movements and empties the catheter bag. Some visits include other chores, such as giving her a bed bath, changing her gown and bed linens, rubbing her limbs with liniment or lotion, or preparing her fortified milk drink. Occasionally, when Mrs. Little asks, she warms up some food, runs by the store to pick up a few items, or stops by a fast-food restaurant. During most visits, Annette sits and talks for awhile, watching the soap operas on the small black and white TV next to Mrs. Little's bed. Periodically she urges Mrs. Little to take her medications and always comes early on clinic days to help her get dressed. Although Annette does not keep abreast of Mrs. Little's regular medical appointments, she does sometimes make her transportation arrangements.

Annette is the worker who sees Mrs. Little most regularly. She worries about her patient's improper nutrition, urging her to eat her home-delivered meals, and monitors her condition. On several occasions she has called her agency to report deterioration in Mrs. Little's health status or to ask advice. Once she called the ambulance to have her hospitalized. Annette deplores the lack of regular care from her patient's family, but, despite her concern and daily visits, she never has assumed a more primary role in Mrs. Little's care. She fills obvious needs and does whatever she is asked to do, but she rarely takes initiative or assumes responsibility for needed managerial tasks. Mrs. Little complains regularly about the services Annette provides, attributing little significance to her caregiving role:

> She's nice, too, her sleepy, TV self. She just can't cook. Says she doesn't know how, and got a husband too. None of them cook as good as I do. Great big fat woman. She always comes late 'cause she don't do nothing. My head nurse said she was supposed to wash my clothes too. She's been putting them under the bed. She don't know how to make up a bed, get the bed all balled up, don't do nothing but mess up the bed. Look how she got my pillow. Got some half-warm water to wash me in.

Janice, the homemaker aide, comes Tuesdays and Thursdays for two hours, increased from the once a week previously scheduled. She generally comes earlier than Annette, but sometimes their visits coincide. While her regular routine includes bringing Mrs. Little breakfast from a fast-food establishment, which she pays for herself, and vacuuming the bedroom and living room, most of her time is spent performing personal care tasks such as bathing Mrs. Little and changing her diaper and bed linens. Sometimes Janice takes it upon herself to do other household chores, like setting mouse traps or organizing Mrs. Little's clothes. When asked, she picks up needed items from the store. Once she bought Mrs. Little's beer. Janice never washes Mrs. Little's clothes, however, nor does she do regular grocery shopping.

Like Annette, Janice entreats Mrs. Little to take her medicine, sometimes successfully, and to eat. She helps her get ready for medical appointments, if they are on a day when she comes, and, once, she called the ambulance when Mrs. Little was having a health crisis. Janice does not monitor Mrs. Little's medical appointments, accompany her to the doctor, or pick up her medicine from County Hospital.

On one occasion, when both aides were together, the two took Mrs. Little out on the front porch. A few times, Janice's little boy, who saves pennies for Mrs. Little, has come with her. Although Janice spends less time with Mrs. Little than Annette, Mrs. Little attaches more significance to her role:

> This young girl that came last Thursday and today, I thought at first, "That's a child," but she sure knew what she was doing.

Cleaned in the living room, too; needed cleaning up, dirty and junky, box with summer rags in it. She got on the ball catching the rats. Came in doing right by me and I was proud of it. God bless her.

At times, though, Janice's role, too, is discredited:

I got the sorriest nurses ever walked on two foots. One supposed to come early, doesn't come till around ten. One in the evening. Neither one do anything, just stand around and talk. Look just alike to me.

## RUBY WASHINGTON

Although Ruby Washington initially had personal care services three times a week, she now receives home health aide visits each weekday. Over the course of this research she has had a variety of aides, who perform services primarily related to personal and health care—assisting with bathing, hair care, medication, and walking, changing bed linens, and taking her vital signs. Mrs. Washington's endorsement of her home care services is tempered by her ready access to Mr. Jones, her husband:

She makes my bed, combs my hair, washes my hair once in a while, gives me my medicine if I haven't had it, puts eye drops in, gives me my bath. I pull off all my clothes. She washes me. I wash my down parts. When she doesn't come, Jones brings me water and sets it on the table. She helps me walk if my legs aren't swollen. One [aide] I had fix the bed, give me my bath, and be ready to go. This nurse is just more cleverer than the others. She talks to me, asks if anything I want done, asks if I take my medicine. She come everyday, but every other day be enough. That's most of the time when I change everything [bed linens]. Jones can give me my eye drops, but she wouldn't have nothing to do if she didn't do that, because when the bed be clean and everything, she won't have to change it but every other day. She do what she know she have to do. I don't have to tell her. She asks me everyday if I need the bed changed. I tell her. Sometimes I do and sometimes I don't. She comb my hair and she say, "You want me to do anything?" She don't hardly have enough to do. I say it's all right. She say it's on account of my blood pressure [that she comes everyday].

## VIOLA WORTH

Viola Worth has a personal care aide, Anne, who comes on Mondays, Wednesdays, and Fridays for two hours. Anne has been with Ms.

Worth for one year. She helps Ms. Worth with her bath, her hair, and dressing and numerous household tasks, including vacuuming, mopping, and dusting, as well as special tasks like washing and ironing curtains, cleaning electric fans, or putting elastic in her pants. Anne is involved in her client's health care, routinely monitoring Ms. Worth's supply of medicine and picking up refills from the pharmacy. She reminds her client about doctor's appointments and once came at 5:30 A.M. to help her prepare for a diagnostic procedure. While Anne has a regular routine for tasks, she is accommodating when Ms. Worth has special needs or prefers to do a job herself. They often sit and talk after Anne finishes her work. Ms. Worth's description of Anne's care clearly indicates the client's own managerial role:

> My main thing is my bath and my medicine, but Anne will do anything I ask her. She dusts, you know. She doesn't dust everyday. She'll more than likely dust tomorrow if I let her, but she may not dust. It's just according [to what is needed]. Maybe if I have something I want her to do extra, I'll say something. I'll say, "You don't have to do so and so 'cause you done this thing that was a little extra for me." But tomorrow, I want to try to think tonight and call her, for I'm going to have to have some medicine. She done already mentioned it, "Now you know you don't want to do without your medicine." I'll have her come about eight-something and have her help me with my bath, like I generally do, and get my medicine. I won't let her do nothing else because she done worked in the field [out of the house] for me.

### REV. JOSEPH SCOTT

For most of the study period, Rev. Scott has had either home health or personal care services four days a week. Usually, the PCA assists with personal care, primarily bathing and helping put on his support hose, does a little cooking, such as putting frozen vegetables on the stove, and sometimes washes a few dishes. When his services switched to Medicare, the care provided by the home health aide (who in this case was the same individual) was more restricted and, in Rev. Scott's view, less valuable.

Because his regular aide, Mrs. Ellis, was promoted from PCA to HHA about the time of the switch to Medicare, Rev. Scott was able to keep her for two years. With the change back to CCSP and the PCA, however, she could no longer be with him. For a few months he had several different personal care aides, who often missed days because of short-staffing at the provider agency.

In addition, Rev. Scott has had three different homemaker aides over the course of the study—two furnished by DFACS and one provided by the CCSP home health agency. The first one, Mrs. Conner, had been with him for over two years until she was transferred to another client. In contrast to the homemaker aide that visits Mrs. Little, the tasks performed by Mrs. Conner, though more limited in scope, had a much more significant role in meeting the caregiving needs of her client. Mrs. Conner came on Wednesdays, usually staying about three hours, and took care of the bulk of Rev. Scott's housekeeping needs. She had a regular routine, which he described:

> Well, she pretty much knows what's to be done. We get laundry done once a month and grocery shopping once a month. I try to space it out so if she gets groceries this week, she'll work at the house next week and then do the laundry next week, so that every other week she'll be where she can do something in the house—to clean or do a little cooking or something like that. Some time if I need any extra things like milk or loaf of bread to make it out for the rest of the month, she'll get that when she goes to the laundry store. She'll pick those up at the store across the street. She have made deposits [at the bank] for me on her way to get groceries. She said she didn't mind.

When Mrs. Conner was transferred, Rev. Scott got a different homemaker. While his new aide had the same routine as Mrs. Conner, she did not accomplish as many tasks, leaving dishes in the sink or failing to put away Rev. Scott's clothes. After several unsuccessful requests for a replacement, Rev. Scott convinced his case manager to change providers—from DFACS to the agency furnishing his CCSP services. Currently, he has the same aide, from the same agency, five days a week. On four days, she provides PCA services for one and a half hours; on the fifth day, she works as an HMA for two hours.

Rev. Scott has experienced highs and lows in service delivery during the years he has received home care services, but his testimony to the value of formal care for him is unequivocal:

> I imagine what things would be like if I weren't getting help. Get up. Get breakfast. Time it takes me to get breakfast and wash dishes, get food for dinner, wash dishes again—no time left. I tried to mop the floor, got tired of it being dirty. Be so tired when night come. Call to get a cab to buy groceries. Sometimes he [the driver] would go inside to help. If I didn't have help getting my clothes. . . .

## LUCY OLIVER

Lucy Oliver's personal care services typically consisted of hair care, which Mr. Oliver cannot do, and occasional assistance with bathing, making the bed, or writing the monthly checks. Since the switch to Medicare, her twice-weekly home health aide services are similar, with the addition of the monitoring of her vital signs.

Although Mr. Oliver can manage many of the personal care tasks aides usually perform, and frequently gives Mrs. Oliver her bath before the aide arrives, they both view the aide's role as a welcome addition to the regular care regimen:

> She's a lot of help. She'll bathe her and put on her clothes, anything she want done. It's really a help because she can't sign checks. They do that for her. I can't write too good. I don't know if she's supposed to do that, but I *can* wash dishes. I'd rather for her to do that [write checks]. It's more important for her to comb her hair than to bathe, but she can do both. All of them are nice. One of them just couldn't plait hair.

## GERALDINE STARR

Geraldine Starr has two homemaker aides—one furnished through CCSP, who comes five days a week for one and one-half hours, and one furnished by the housing authority, who is scheduled to come once a week for an unspecified amount of time. At the beginning of this study, she also had both senior companion and home health aide services under Medicare, but they have since terminated. [Although a senior companion technically does not belong under one of the aide classifications, her care will be included because of the similarity in the kinds of services performed.]

While her senior companion, Lois, was with Mrs. Starr, she took care of many ADL, IADL, and health care tasks, including some Mrs. Starr was able to do herself. Eventually she even assumed a primary and managerial role. Lois came four or five days a week, usually arriving around 9:00 A.M. and staying till 2:00 or 3:00 P.M. She planned menus, shopped, cooked, cleaned, washed clothes, directed other formal workers, and communicated with informal helpers. Lois monitored Mrs. Starr's health care regimen, including keeping up with her many medicines and assisting her in taking them correctly. She summoned help in emergencies and handled many business matters. She also frequently called Mrs. Starr at night and on the weekends to remind her to take her medicine and often brought her little gifts. Mrs. Starr became quite attached to Lois and often praised the way she performed her many tasks:

> I wouldn't want nobody better than her. She sure do keep the floors clean, bed clothes white as snow. Nobody can make up a bed like Lois.

The home health aide, Myrtice, came twice a week. Her typical services were related to personal care and health care, including assisting Mrs. Starr with bathing, rubbing her with liniment, and taking her vital signs. On one visit, which lasted an hour, Myrtice bathed Mrs. Starr's feet, rubbed her with lotion, weighed her, and took her vital signs. Mrs. Starr attributed little significance to her role:

> Myrtice is the big, stout, dark one. She bathes me, rubs my legs down, listens to my heart. She's just a nurse's aide, no guarantee of a nurse.

The homemaker aide, Vicky, who has been with Mrs. Starr over the entire course of the research period, now comes five days a week for one and a half hours. She usually comes in the afternoon, anytime from 3:00 P.M. on, and performs a variety of personal care, housekeeping, and health care tasks, not necessarily on a regular basis. These include assisting with bathing, dressing, and hair care, washing clothes, cleaning, cooking, shopping, going to the bank, and changing the bed. On one visit Vicky emptied the garbage, swept the floor, and sat and talked. Another day, she helped Mrs. Starr get ready to go to the doctor, fixed her breakfast, and pushed her downstairs to wait for her transportation. Vicky always arranges her schedule to accommodate Mrs. Starr's trips to her doctor and the bank and once in a while picks up groceries on the weekends. Like Mrs. Little's homemaker aide, Vicky does no regular cooking or shopping, even with daily visits. Although clearly fond of Vicky, Mrs. Starr was at first complimentary but later more critical of her work and the value of her services, frequently comparing her to Lois:

> She's very sweet, quite young. I wish you could see how she cleaned my stove yesterday. She stayed with me a good little bit yesterday, plaited my hair. I didn't let her wash my clothes. She does pretty good. She cleans good . . . . That child ain't able, another young one, poor critter. She has two young children. She comes 'way in the evening. Sits up there and go to sleep. They just ain't going to do

the way you think they do. Vicky didn't half mop. Lois used to put Clorox on the floor. Somedays they come and do little or nothing, empty the garbage.

In addition to her other aides, Mrs. Starr also has a homemaker aide, Pat, furnished weekly by the housing authority. Some weeks she does not come and often switches her day, but her regular chores are washing Mrs. Starr's bed linens and picking up her food stamps.

## SALLY FINCH

Sally Finch has two kinds of aides—a personal care aide, furnished by CCSP, who comes three times a week for one hour, and a homemaker aide from DFACS, who comes every other Wednesday. Her personal care aide has changed numerous times since the start of this research. Brenda, who had the longest term of any one aide, stayed six months. After Brenda left, Mrs. Finch has not had a regular aide. Her homemaker aide from DFACS, Martha, however, until a recent change, had been with her for two years.

Mrs. Finch's PCA services are restricted to personal care, such as assisting with her bath, dressing, and hair care, cleaning up in the bathroom, and changing the bed. Her homemaker aide attends strictly to housekeeping tasks—laundry, defrosting the refrigerator, any heavy cleaning that Mrs. Finch cannot do, and sometimes mixing a batch of cornbread batter, since Mrs. Finch has difficulty stirring. Although Mrs. Finch used to let Martha pay her telephone bill, she is reluctant as yet to trust the new aide with her money.

Mrs. Finch appreciates her aides's caregiving roles:

> I love it [having her come]. Now, I could put my things in the washer, but about folding 'em up and all that, I couldn't do it, and about going to the shower, I couldn't, because I cannot wash my back and my head.

She feels that they meet her day-to-day needs, but wishes aides still were allowed to accompany her to County Hospital for her clinic visits, in her view her most urgent caregiving need:

> Going to the doctor is what I'm having trouble with now. I need somebody to go with me. When you get to the hospital, they don't have people to help you. I need someone to push me around. Now, Kate [a former aide] used to go with me everywhere I had to go.

\* \* \* \* \*

The role of home care aide can be quite pivotal in the long-term caregiving scheme, providing the bulk of necessary care, or it can serve a less consequential role. How it plays out for each of these clients depends on a series of conditions and events related both to the client and to the aide, including the recognition of a need by the worker and the client, the action by the aide in response to that awareness, and the client's acceptance of the needed service. Some aides assume an expanded role, and some do less than is expected, but it is clear that the client sometimes exerts significant control over the caregiving process.

In the following chapters we find out what these differences in the care from aides mean to the clients, and we explore some of the factors that influence the effectiveness of the formal caregiving system. The focus again will be on the care from aides. These data show—as did those concerning our informants' informal caregiving experiences—that each care recipient, with her or his unique beliefs and values, personalities, abilities, and lifetimes of experiences, plays a major role in the outcome.

## REFERENCES

1. N. N. Eustis, R. A. Kane, and L. R. Fischer, Home Care Quality and the Home Care Worker: Beyond Quality Assurance as Usual, *The Gerontologist, 33*:1, pp. 64-73, 1993.
2. J. F. Gubrium and A. Sankar (eds.), *The Home Care Experience*, Sage Publications, Inc., Newbury Park, California, 1990.
3. M. Cantor and E. Chichin, *Stress and Strain Among Home Care Workers of the Frail Elderly*, Brookdale Research Institute on Aging, Third Age Center, Fordham University, New York, 1990.
4. N. N. Eustis and L. R. Fischer, Relationships Between Home Care Clients and Their Workers: Implications for Quality of Care, *The Gerontologist, 31*:4, pp. 447-456, 1991.

# CHAPTER
# 9

# Quality of Care—The Client's Reality

*There's some of them good. Some of them get paid but need training.*
*Don't send anybody that don't know how to do. Heap of 'em know*
*and won't. Not supposed to hire nobody that don't know how to do,*
*didn't even know how to make a bed. It burns me up.*

Sally Finch

The rapid growth of the home care industry has prompted increased public and congressional concern with the quality of community-based care [1-5]. Although little data are available about home care, reports of bad care have become more numerous, many focusing on paraprofessional workers [6]. Problems cited include physical abuse, theft, financial exploitation, deficiencies in basic knowledge, tardiness, failure to show up or spend the specified amount of time, insensitivity, disrespect, and intimidation [1, 3, 4, 6]. Because of difficulties with recruitment and retention, rapid turnover also is a widespread problem [7-9]. In addition to personnel problems, the whole service delivery system is often charged with being fragmented and irrational [5].

Most information about home care comes from evaluations of the numerous community-based demonstration projects, which focus primarily on outcomes of care, such as cost-effectiveness, mortality, functional abilities, unmet needs, and client satisfaction [6, 11-13]. Little research has addressed the *processes* of care—what is done to and for a client, by whom, and in what manner—and how they relate to quality. Rarely is the client's perspective sought [14]. Only minimal information is available about how often clients perceive that the worker's personality or work style is a problem or whether problems stem from workers' performance or the way their jobs are defined [6].

In this chapter, we examine the ways these seven African-American clients define and evaluate the care received. While they have

169

differences in specific preferences for how they want to be helped, they share many attitudes and values about which aspects of the caregiving process are most important to them and about the quality of care.

We found that they care a great deal about job performance. On the whole, clients want aides to be competent and diligent, to take initiative, and to do those tasks that are most salient, in the manner that is favored. They prefer that aides come at convenient times, which usually means in the morning, and on their regularly scheduled days. Unless a problem arises, these clients prefer to have continuity in caregivers.

Clients care equally, and often more strongly, about an aide's work style, personality, and attitudes toward them as individuals and toward personal job performance. Clients want to be treated with kindness, gentleness, and respect as human beings whose opinions and preferences matter. The manifestations of these various caregiving traits help clients define aides into two groups—those who care about their work and their clients and perform their tasks willingly and those who do not. Which of these two categories their aides belong to influences how these clients feel about themselves as recipients of care and how they evaluate the quality of care received.

Other research suggests that many of these attitudes are not unique to these particular clients or to African-American clients. Kate Quinton, the old woman of Irish descent described so vividly by journalist Sheehan, was more likely to overlook shortcomings in job performance when her home care workers had "willing" attitudes [9]. When workers took pride in their own efforts or adopted more expanded roles, testimonies of their regard for her, she was happier, and her health and functional ability even showed signs of improvement.

Eustis and Fischer conducted in-depth interviews with home care clients in rural and urban Minnesota and found most complaints about quality of care concerned, not job performance, but lack of sensitivity or caring on the part of the provider [14]. These respondents also stressed the importance of the need for flexibility both in range of task and in scheduling, emphasizing a preference for individualized services—services that they both want and need. Carlsson-Agren and colleagues emphasized the need to consider clients' personal timetables when scheduling visits in order to preserve their highest level of autonomy [15]. Eustis and her co-workers also reported on data compiled from home care client focus groups that emphasized the importance of workers having caring attitudes toward their clients [6].

A survey of home care providers and consumers in Maryland provided further evidence of clients' concerns about the aspects of care that relate more to their general civil rights and protections and their nonmedical quality of life than to the more clinical events of care [16]. These quality of life concerns were exemplified by rights such as "respect for property," which was rated by 90 percent of clients as very important. An example given by the authors was the client who did not want to remove the handmade throw rug that had been next to her bed for the last twenty years. Maintaining the "normalcy" of their personal space, their home, and their day-to-day lifestyle was the primary client concern.

Research involving nursing home residents suggests many similarities with home care clients. A report compiled by the National Citizens' Coalition for Nursing Home Reform [17] identified treatment with dignity and respect and a caring attitude as crucial elements of quality care.

Although the seven clients reported on here share many concerns about what constitutes good care, some contradictions are apparent, even within an individual. As was so clearly evident in their relationships with informal caregivers, these contradictory values stem largely from the quest for self-reliance as it clashes with the reality of dependence. We see Geraldine Starr wanting to take care of her own needs and not wanting "to bother with any of them," yet longing to feel cared for. We see her having great difficulty giving herself a bath, yet resenting her aides who try to help. Lustbader found similar paradoxes among the ill and disabled people she studied [18]. She noted that with increased loss of independence, people become more torn by contradictory urges. "When success at even ordinary tasks becomes elusive, some people resent being rescued as much as they want desperately to be spared their frustrations" [18, p. 123]. The tendency of clients like Mrs. Starr and Mrs. Little to be chronic complainers or to lash out at their caregivers may be attempts to assert their independence or to gain power by demeaning the abilities of the workers they depend on.

We see these same frustrations in the inconsistent biases of some clients for aides to perform their tasks without having to be asked or instructed, yet performing them according to clients' personal specifications, preferably the way they would do them if able; in the preference for aides to be thorough and to do a job "right," while recognizing, and not superseding, clients' own potential roles. Part of the problem rests in the difficulties clients have in admitting their needs for help in doing tasks they have always done—and would still prefer to do—independently. As Lustbader so aptly put it, "to accept help is to miss a chance to prevail, and to go on struggling is taxing and upsetting" [18, p. 123].

## MEASURING GOOD CARE

*. . . how they treat you and the way they go along about their job.*
Viola Worth

Each of these African American elders has specific attitudes about, and expectations for, the processes of formal care. These include attitudes about what, when, how, and even if tasks should be performed, who should perform them, and how caregivers should present themselves during the caregiving process. Some beliefs are shared by all of these individuals, while others are unique to particular clients. In all cases these attitudes and expectations affect the caregiving process, sometimes in quite unexpected ways. In her words above, Ms. Worth identifies those aspects of care deemed most important by these clients: "How they treat you and how they go along about their job."

### Job Performance

Each of these clients prefers that aides be competent, that they "know how to do." As noted in previous discussions, the women in this study have always kept their own houses, and for all, except Mrs. Washington, domestic work was their primary work role. It is not surprising they have knowledge of, and distinct preferences about, how household jobs should be performed. The meaning of competence for them has emerged from their own past experiences and often relates to techniques they themselves once used. As Geraldine Starr expresses in her critique of Vicky's care, "the right way," is the way she cleaned for herself and for other people:

> I don't feel good enough that I can come behind you and clean. I tell Vicky the same thing. She pull something out and just leave it, moved the mop out of the bathroom, put it in the pantry. I just wish I was able to tend to things myself. I was taught to do things right. If I was able, I wouldn't be bothered with none of them.

Like Mrs. Starr, each of these clients often defines the "right" and competent way as her or his *own* way. Ms. Worth's impassioned judgment of a former aide's reluctance to follow her directions, in this instance for fixing her hair, gives explicit evidence that some clients believe they have the right to control their territories, be it their houses or their heads:

> This is *my* head! She got her little way, like she don't want to do what *you* want her to do.

When aides conform to "the client's way," they give clients feelings of greater power and a more credible role-identity—as one who knows the "right" way.

As a rule, these clients like aides to use their allotted time to do needed chores, not tend to their own business or "do nothing." Viola Worth regularly praises Anne for her diligence, a trait she sees in herself, yet was critical of a former aide who many times began her day on the telephone:

> I've had some that looked like they didn't want to do nothing but sit down. Anne works more like me than anybody else. Anne believes in getting things done. She comes in and goes to work. She works like it's her last day. Trisha put her work behind to tend to her own business, putting off her job for doing nothing. I get upset with her. You ain't hurtin' nobody but yourself if you don't do right.

Mrs. Starr also complained about an aide who, upon arriving at her apartment, would sit down and fill out service forms and call clients she was to visit later in the day:

> First thing, she sits down and does paperwork and then gets on my phone. *I* can't use the phone. She used the phone more that I did.

One aide confirmed how other workers sometimes do not do what they are "supposed to do":

> She [one of her clients] say the aides, when they were there, they was always on the phone or something, and they never had time for *her*. They didn't do what they were supposed to do. But I got her house straight. Her bathroom was so filthy, I was even scared to walk *into* the bathroom. I got that house looking good, and I cleaned and I cleaned and I cleaned, and it looks like that today. The lady she has now keeps it up for her.

Taking initiative is another trait commonly valued in aides, as expressed by Ms. Worth, who prefers that aides not always wait for directions, but rather anticipate her needs:

> I like for them to go on about their business with me not having to tell them. They know what they supposed to do. Unless we ask them to do something extra, go on and do what they supposed to do. Come in and say good morning and see about me and then go do what they doing.

Mrs. Finch, too, appreciates this trait:

> Come in, help you with your bath and then [do] anything they see.
> You don't have to ask them. They go in there, and, if there are dirty
> dishes in the sink, they wash them up. Your bed need making, they
> make your bed, then your bathroom, and then, if you want them to
> cook some breakfast, they fix it. And she would do it. I never did
> have to ask her to do one thing.

We found that client viewpoints about job performance interact with
other attitudes. We will see in Chapter 11 that the preference for
initiative is reinforced by the difficulties clients experience in requesting and directing help. Because of her near-total dependence, Mrs.
Little particularly appreciates not having to ask for help:

> Don't ask, "Do you want me to bathe you?" Go on and do what you
> have to do and get it over with. They supposed to look and see. She
> [one aide] didn't even ask if I had an action [bowel movement].
> When that girl [her homemaker aide, Janice] came in here this
> morning, after she asked me how I am, first thing she do is throw
> the covers back [to check if she had a bowel movement]. There's
> some nice girls and boys; there some mean girls and boys. She's
> supposed to see about these without my telling her.

Sometimes, however, the goal of the care receiver to retain control
over the caregiving process or to emphasize self-reliance takes
precedence over the preference for the aide's taking initiative. The
ascendancy of this attitude accounts for the times when Ms. Worth
wishes Anne would *not* just "go on about her business" but, rather,
would wait for Ms. Worth to direct her. By waiting for instruction,
Anne shows she recognizes Ms. Worth's role in caregiving and her
competence as a homemaker:

> She's gonna do like she want to do anyway. I say lots Anne do, don't
> have to be done everyday. Ain't no need in running the vacuum
> every time. I don't have nobody running in and out of here. I love
> my clean, but there ain't no need in her mopping back there all
> three days. I mopped Saturday. She's going over my work, and the
> floor ain't dirty.

When Mrs. Starr began to feel that her companion, Lois, was assuming
too much control—taking over areas of care that she considered beyond
the realm of an appropriate role—she too rebelled:

She worries too much about things that are not her concern—going down and tellin' folks about my business. I don't like anybody throwing my business around. I just don't like her changing my business. I want to go out and get my money myself. She was going to make my rent receipt out. I buy mine at the bank. I tend to my business myself. She went through that folder [from the home health agency] and told Myrtice [the home health aide] what she was supposed to do. Lord'll put a stop to her mouth if she run that little red thing too much!

Like informal caregivers, the aides who help these clients often must walk a thin line if they are to satisfy them.

## Time

Time is an important construct in a client's view of services—the time aides come, the amount of time they stay, and their use of time. Personal care and homemaker aides who provide services through CCSP are allotted a maximum of two hours to perform their work in one client's home, since these types of aides usually serve four to five clients per day. Homemaker aides furnished by DFACS generally visit only two clients a day and are allowed to stay for approximately three hours. Home health aides stay the amount of time necessary to complete the job, with the expectation that forty-five minutes to an hour is sufficient. They generally serve eight to ten clients per day, sometimes as many as fifteen.

We saw in Chapter 4 that these clients have daily routines. Obviously, with the number of clients that aides serve, the client's preference for scheduling visits cannot always be accommodated, but it is important that formal services not upset their personal routines. Each of these participants prefers that aides come in the morning. The primary reason is that, once bathed and dressed, they can get on with their day, as Ms. Worth explains:

If they're going to be after 12:00, they might as well stay away. That gets on my nerves. If I want to go somewhere, my girl done turnt me loose [made her scheduled visit].

Even though she rarely leaves her apartment, Mrs. Finch too likes to have her aide come early:

I love that. I be the first one, so I can dress and do what I want to do, don't be sitting around in my night clothes.

For Mrs. Starr, morning care is more useful because morning is when she is at her weakest and in need of more help:

> I asked them to send her in the morning. That's my hardest time. Fix me a little breakfast. This kitchen is tearing me up. In the morning is my weakest time. By twelve or one o'clock, I kind of spruce up.

In addition to their preferences for morning service, some clients have the perception that aides cannot perform services as well in the afternoon, particularly when it is late. This perception is based on their observations of aides' behavior, as Mrs. Starr notes:

> Vicky came in so late Friday she couldn't do too much. That child ain't able. She comes 'way in the evening—sits up there and go to sleep. They just ain't gonna do the way you think they do.

Rev. Scott made a similar observation about one aide who typically arrived late:

> She came in here about four o'clock and act like she had run out of gas. Sit down for a few minutes and act like she don't want to get up.

Rev. Scott likes his aide to come in the morning, but for him it is also critical to know *when* a worker is coming, so that he can plan his day:

> Well, it's important if I know about what time they coming like, uh, if I know if they coming around noon or shortly after, I can get out in the yard or the sunshine. I might not hear the phone if they call before they come. I prefer they come after 9:30. Give me a chance to do little things I have to do and maybe get breakfast. I always thought it would be better to get it over with before the afternoon. Then I have the afternoons free. I try not to be too choicy on that. They have other patients. I understand that some they have to go early enough to help with breakfast.

For Rev. Scott, a regular schedule is preferable to having aides call before they come, which is the official protocol. This arrangement gives him more control over his day, and having to stay close to the phone to await the call is an added burden. Mrs. Starr also prefers that aides not call before coming. Getting to the phone can be a slow and frustrating process, particularly if she is in the bathroom. Anyway, she finds it unnecessary since she is almost always at home:

They *know* I can't go nowhere!

The amount of time aides remain in a client's home can influence a client's perception of the success or failure of the care provided. For home health aides, whose time is most limited, a common client perception is that aides are rushed and do not have sufficient time. This viewpoint is not necessarily related to whether all necessary tasks are accomplished. When Mrs. Starr had home health services, she frequently complained that her aide's visits were too short:

> She just run in here yesterday and running out. Had to go get her child and put me last. Just long enough to give me a fly bath. Ready to fly out the door.

Mrs. Little had a similar reaction to the time spent by her home health aide:

> Ain't got time to wash my face and hands. Just come in and sit down and ask how I am. I tell you she ain't got time, and better not let me go to sleep, [or] she's gone.

On the other hand, her view of her homemaker aide, who stays at least two hours, contrasts significantly:

> She stays here all day and all night.

Such viewpoints are based on the client's observations of the actions of their aides and on how clients define the amount of time required to perform a particular job adequately. Once again this definition often derives from their own housekeeping experiences. Mrs. Starr explains how good cleaning and cooking demand time:

> Don't do nothing [the aide]. I used to keep it clean. Kept it jam up. Take me a whole half a day to clean. . . . She ain't the best of cooks. She ain't got *time* for it.

Clients differ in what they consider the optimum length for an aide's visit. For the most part, this view is based on the individual's own preferences and need for services. According to Mrs. Finch, once the job is done, the aide is free to leave, even if the time spent is less that authorized. She believes the aide *should* leave if she is not "doin' something." Ms. Worth, too, does not always require the full two hours of service, particularly if an aide is diligent, and it is Ms. Worth's choice:

Anne don't sit and talk. She comes in and goes to work. If she finishes, I tell her to go on.

For clients with greater needs, however, an aide's leaving early usually is defined as problematic. Rev. Scott expressed dissatisfaction with an aide who regularly left early before completing the necessary tasks:

She mops the floor and starts walking. She doesn't even look at the dirty dishes in the sink.

## Regularity of Services

Sometimes aides do not come on the days that they are scheduled. These absences occur in varying degrees and for a variety of reasons, some more legitimate than others. Holidays interrupt regularly scheduled visits, as do various personal problems, such as sickness or lack of child care. Occasionally, aides just do not show up, and clients are unaware of the reason or even that they are not coming until late in the day. Lack of communication also can cause aides to miss visits, as when Mrs. Little failed to notify the agency she was home from the hospital and in need of services.

In cases of expected absences the client frequently is notified directly by the aide or the agency, but not always. Sometimes aides fail to notify the agency when absent, and, because of inadequate staff, agencies do not always have extra workers to send. In some instances clients choose not to have replacement workers. Whether or not clients define these absences as problematic depends on their alternatives. When Ms. Worth's aide misses a day, or even a week, as a rule she does not view the absence as a problem because she can manage many basic daily tasks herself:

I'm one of them that can make it. There are some that just *need*.

Other participants like Mrs. Washington and Mrs. Oliver have informal caregivers who can fill in. The severity of the hardship imposed also depends on when the absence occurs. When Rev. Scott's homemaker aide failed to come on his routine laundry day, her absence was not a problem, but when she missed the day set aside for monthly grocery shopping, his need was severe. Another time, when his personal care aide left the agency and the agency delayed in finding a replacement, he had no aide services for ten days. During this period, he had difficulty meeting basic needs.

For Mrs. Little, the absence of an aide is always a problem. The gaps in services over weekends already create hardships for her, and if additional absences occur on a Friday or Monday, as sometimes happens with holidays, her needs are compounded. Although agencies attempt to send replacements in cases of severe need, they often do not have sufficient resources.

## Continuity of Care

Aide turnover was a variable problem. Mrs. Washington had five different aides during the twelve-month study period, while Ms. Worth, Mrs. Starr, and Mrs. Little experienced minimal changes. Each person, however, expressed a preference for having continuous care from the same aide, particularly a well-liked aide like Mrs. Oliver's aide, Sarah:

> I don't know why they change so often. Say everything is fine and then they up and change. I liked Sarah. I wished she'd come. Get somebody you like and then they take 'em.

One reason given by several clients for this preference was the familiarity that develops between client and caregiver over long-term associations. Mrs. Starr, characteristically hard-to-please, is able to tolerate some of Vicky's undesirable traits because she is "used to" her:

> Vicky said she'd be coming everyday for the same amount of time. She'll probably run me crazy, but I'm used to Vicky. I likes her so much because I'm so well acquainted with her. I ain't in any shape to learn another one.

Having a regular aide eases the burden of both giving and receiving care, as Rev. Scott states:

> Well, it means alot. A person that comes regular knows what supposed to be done, where things are. That takes a lot off of me. Coming in new, have to show them everything, tell where to go. It takes a while to kind of learn where everything is. I don't know. It just makes it better for somebody to come kind of regular.

Continuity of aides can also lead to a more expanded aide role. In most cases, some degree of continuity was necessary to build trust, especially enough trust for clients to allow aides to handle their money. Although Mrs. Finch lets her homemaker, who has been with her for two years, pay her telephone bill, she is reluctant to trust her personal care aides, who change frequently:

> Every time I look around I got a new one. Can't trust 'em with your money. They might not come back.

As we will see in Chapter 10, keeping the same aide for an extended period of time can foster the development of close socio-emotional ties between clients and their aides, as Ms. Worth pointed out about her relationship with Anne:

> They let her stay with me so long she was just like family. She come to be just part of me.

## Treatment of Clients

> *I can get along with any of them as long as they treat me right.*
> Sally Finch

How one is treated by formal aides is of utmost importance to these seven clients, sometimes more important than the actual care they receive. Treatment here encompasses the manner in which caregivers interact with clients while providing care as well as the attitudes they have toward their clients and toward their roles as caregivers and the work they do.

In her ten years of receiving help, Viola Worth has found that some aides scored better than others in this area. She is forever praising Anne's kind ways but complained about a new RN who did not exhibit such traits:

> That's a sweet lady. God sent me you and Anne. She's real nice to me. Some people in the field [home care] don't need to be in it. Some are more gentler than others, just their nature. You don't want somebody that's just going come in and look at you if they supposed to wait on you personal, like your bath and everything. Just be kind to one another.

Mrs. Little, too, appreciates the kindness of her aide, Janice, whose manner contrasts with that of her other aide, Annette:

> She's mighty nice, the one that comes on Thursday. God bless her, someone to take an interest in you. Takes good pains with me. Wants to rub my legs with lotion, keeps from being so chapped up. Always bring me something. She'll warm up food for me. She's real

nice. Got mother wit in her bones, helping the poor and the sick. I appreciate all that.

Mr. Oliver agrees that the manner in which a service is offered often takes priority over how the work is performed, and a pleasing personality is an added bonus:

> Everybody like Sarah. She make you like her. One thing, she has a nice personality. That goes a long way. She's *real* nice. Sometime you can meet people and it seems like you been knowing them all your life. It's a lot in the way people talk to you. She fixed hair good too. If you like somebody, that counts more than anything. All of them have did their job. Like this ambulance [transportation service], I called two or three, and they were telling me like I should already know. This lady is so *nice*, we take them no matter how long we have to wait. It must be their policy for people in the company to treat everybody right. When you treated nice, you get that back.

Good treatment also means showing respect for clients, for their belongings, their privacy, their ways of doing things, their own roles as caregivers, and, most importantly, their right to self-determination.

Often this means seeing clients as individuals with unique abilities and needs and respecting their right to make choices about their care. When Lois tried to "measure" Mrs. Starr's self-care efforts by those of other clients, Mrs. Starr became quite angry:

> I got tired of hearing that—telling me about people older than me doing for theyselves, fixing their own breakfast. I've had a hard sickness. If you don't want to do it, just go on. Throwing up to me about how somebody else doing, "You just don't try." I'm not gonna get all that strength she's talking about. I ask the Lord to give me strength if He wants to. Man ain't gonna do it. She tries to measure people by other people. Ain't no two people alike.

Lois's unsolicited advice, her exhortations to try even harder, are misinterpreted by Mrs. Starr as an unwillingness to help and as attempts to control her behavior. In Mrs. Starr's view, Lois did not understand that she was trying as hard as she could, but in her *own* way.

Mrs. Starr also objected to the way one aide "fussed" at her, in this case for not taking a shower:

> She put me in that old shower. [Her apartment only has a shower.] I ain't never cared for showers. I need to get in a tub and soak

myself. "Go home and stay and don't come back! I just don't like your attitude. I ain't used to anybody fussin' at me. *I* do the fussin', not you."

Mrs. Starr has devised her own way of bathing (using a wash basin and rag), and she remembers that a County doctor once cautioned her that taking a shower might cause her to suffer another stroke. Firmly set in her ways and her beliefs, Mrs. Starr is only frustrated by this aide's particular style of helping.

Mrs. Little, also characteristically resistent, responded in a similar manner to Annette's pleas to improve her self-care:

> Some people get on your nerves. You doin' all you can, and some-body come along and tell you what to do. She didn't do nothing but tell me what to say and not say, do and not do. I want one that got good sense to help me and not try to tear me down. I'm hand-icapped, and I ain't gonna try. I don't try to tell nobody how they feel 'cause I don't know. I don't know nobody's feelings. I don't know if they can help do anything or not. They don't have to be beggin'.

Although Mrs. Little often tries to be self-reliant, her actions are of her own choosing, and her typical non-compliance is one of her few remain-ing choices.

Efforts of formal workers to educate clients about such matters as diet or exercise were interpreted as attempts to control, or as disrespect for clients' own knowledge. Mrs. Finch explains her preference for an aide who does not try to "teach" her:

> She's a good person too—don't try to teach you. Some try to teach you, think you don't know any better. Catherine [a former aide], she thought she was my mama, just bossing, "You ain't got no business doing that, not with your blood pressure." I don't like too much bossin' now that I've gotten older.

Neither do clients like aides to assume a motherly attitude, relegat-ing them to child-like status. Mrs. Starr expressed this view in her usual forthright manner:

> She asks you like you some kind of child. I ain't no child! She wants to be your mama, and I'm way older than she is. I'm old enough to be her great-grandmother.

Clients appreciate aides who respect their personal space, their belongings, and their privacy. This can mean not throwing away things too quickly while cleaning, a complaint Mrs. Little has about her half-sister, Marion, as well as her homemaker aide:

> That housekeeping woman, she'll throw away anything if she gets a chance. She says, "You have more junk." Well, I likes it.

It means being careful about clients' limited resources, a frequent worry of Mrs. Starr:

> She puts too much soap on the rag. She's wasteful. I had to buy three bars of soap, she had so much soap on my skin. I had to argue about the nitroglycerin pads. I don't wet them. I wash around them. I can only get so many each month from Medicaid. That child picked up a bag of them Depends. They was too thin. I don't have that kind of money to waste. She thought she had the right thing, instead of being sure, but I straightened her out. I told her, I said, "Look honey, I don't have but one little check, and when that money goes out of my hand, it doesn't go back into my hand no more. I try to stretch it as far as I can. Then, you don't walk in a store and just pick up something and walk out with it."

It means not being too nosy or meddlesome, another frequent concern of Mrs. Starr:

> She's all the time ramblin' in the closet, opening the drawers, looking in the refrigerator, turning on the television. She kept asking me for things, wanted everything she see. Just things to flusterate me, mix my mind all up.

And it means being trustworthy, treatment Rev. Scott appreciated from his homemaker aide, Mrs. Conner:

> She seem to be a nice person. She said on one occasion she didn't want to take anything from me, she'd rather give me something. She had gone to the grocery store, and it happened that she got shorted on groceries. Well, she went back out there, and they gave her the groceries. She wanted me to know she wasn't trying to cheat me out of anything.

From the viewpoints of these seven clients, the formal caregivers' attitudes toward them as clients are reflected in the attitudes they have toward their jobs—whether they care about the quality of care they provide and their willingness to provide the care clients prefer. In the preceding discussion of job performance, clients often accounted for performance in terms of an aide's *desire* to do a good job. In the discussion of the role of aides, it was evident that some aides assumed a more expanded role than others—did more than was required or expected of them.

Rev. Scott accounts for these differences in terms of the degree of pride that aides have in their work:

> Some people take more pride in their work than others. See this wrinkly shirt I have on. Mrs. Conner [his former HMA] wouldn't have done that. She would have taken a rack to put them on when they came out of the dryer so the wrinkles would fall out. I think it depends on the individual whether they have any pride in their job or not.

Mr. Oliver agrees:

> Some have that *attitude*. Some just waitin' on their paycheck. Some take an interest in their work. I guess if all of us were the same, we wouldn't have to pray.

One of Mrs. Finch's aides, Brenda, who regularly assumed an expanded role, taking gifts to her clients and performing extra chores, explained that a fundamental facet of her job is caring about the old people for whom she provides services:

> Some people do it for the money, *just* for the money. I do it because I like it. I *love* old people. One lady asked me, "Why do you always be hugging on my grandmother?" and I say, "Because I *love* your grandmother."

Mrs. Little's home health aide, Annette, described her motivations similarly:

> Some people go right in, give a bath, take pulse, temperature, respiration, "Sign right here." How you gonna know how they feel? I should be able to say, "She's not eating well, has a stomach virus, leg not getting better." I call my job and let 'em know, "I think you need to get somebody out to help." Other girls don't care if they live or die. Everybody got a purpose in the world, reason to be alive. I'm just here to take care of you. If you're greedy, you want to go for the money. It's for the care of the patient. These folks need help.

As we emphasized in Chapter 7, a willing and caring attitude on the part of an informal caregiver can reduce the emotional costs of receiving care. The same is true in interactions with formal caregivers. As expressed in the words of Rev. Scott, aides' attitudes about their jobs affect not only how the work is done but also how these clients feel about themselves:

> Some have a desire to be helpful to the people they serve moreso than others. Some more concerned about making the time and getting on about. Others seem to care enough about their job to make sure they've done what they're supposed to. It is the service, but maybe a service that could be better. Some things are essential for them to do. It might be done by somebody that has a pleasant attitude, but still it gets done. Some people are more willing to do. It makes a difference in how you feel.

Because Rev. Scott has few alternatives for caregivers and is dependent in many ways, any service is valuable to him, but it is easier for him to accept his dependency if the care provider has a caring and willing attitude.

The kindness shown by Mrs. Little's homemaker aide, Janice, also lessens her client's emotional distress:

> She's kind, just as kind as can be. I said, "I'm sorry I'm so messed up." [She replied,] "Why you're sorry? I'm sent here to clean you up. If I have to stay all day with you, I'll stay. I'll clean you up like you should be."

Janice's understanding of Mrs. Little's feelings in this situation—an understanding which she communicates to her client during the caregiving process—makes the humiliating experience of having her diaper changed less damaging to Mrs. Little's self-image.

Yet, as we found in informal caregiving relationships, some formal caregivers demonstrate via their actions an undeniable reluctance to help. Mrs. Starr attributes this type of behavior to her aide, Vicky, and it is clear that her disabilities render her ill-equipped to withstand Vicky's recalcitrant attitude:

> Vicky's got some funny ways too. She'll get mad right quick. Say something, and she'll make a funny face. I can't stand for her to act like she don't want to do it, turn up her nose, "I'll get that the next day. Haven't got time today." I don't want no argument. If I have to argue with them, I'd rather for them to just go on. I haven't got that kind of strength. I don't need somebody with an attitude.

Such unwilling demeanor also adversely affects clients' emotional states. Mrs. Washington, who feels powerless in her dependency, poignantly describes her experience with an unwilling aide:

> She act like she don't want to do the job, do one thing and ready to go. Don't fix the bed good. Ask to sign before she finish. It hurts my feelings when they talk like that. I takes [put up with] a lot because I can't help myself.

* * * * *

These data show that what happens during the process of care is crucial to how these clients define care quality. It is also clear that much of what these clients want in terms of desirable outcomes—to feel cared about and afforded the right to dignity, respect, and some degree of self-determination—depends on the caregiving process. We would apply to home care Berwick and Knapp's [19] dictum about health care in general: ". . . what healthcare delivers is not outcome—in the sense of improved longevity or function—but rather process, itself." In providing quality care, aides often are called upon to have the sensitivity and insight of trained psychologists, as well as the patience of Job. Those who succeed do so by gaining an understanding of their clients and of their own personal definitions of good care.

In the following chapter we will explore the socio-emotional aspects of the formal caregiving experience, focusing on the meaning of social interactions and on the nature of interpersonal relationships that develop between clients and aides.

## REFERENCES

1. H. Weiss, Quality of Care: Bringing it into the Community, *Contemporary LTC*, pp. 24-26, 1987.
2. P. Doty, K. Liu, and J. Wiener, An Overview of Long-Term Care, *Health Care Financing Review, 6*, pp. 69-78, 1985.
3. N. Mumma, Quality and Cost Control of Home Care Services Through Coordinated Funding, *QRB, 17*, pp. 271-278, 1987.
4. C. Harrington, Quality Access and Costs: Public Policy and Home Health Care, *Nursing Outlook, 36*, pp. 164-166, 1988.
5. C. Harrington and L. A. Grant, The Delivery, Regulation, and Politics of Home Care: A California Case Study, *The Gerontologist, 30*:4, pp. 451-461, 1990.
6. N. N. Eustis, R. A. Kane, and L. R. Fischer, Home Care Quality and the Home Care Worker: Beyond Quality Assurance as Usual, *The Gerontologist, 33*:1, pp. 64-73, 1993.

7. P. Feldman, Work Life Improvements for Home Care Workers: Impact and Feasibility, *The Gerontologist, 33*:1, pp. 47-54, 1993.
8. M. MacAdam, Home Care Reimbursement and Effects on Personnel, *The Gerontologist, 33*:1, pp. 55-63, 1993.
9. S. Sheehan, *Kate Quinton's Days*, New American Library, New York, 1984.
10. P. Kemper, R. Brown, G. Carcagno, R. Applebaum, J. Christianson, W. Carson, S. Dunstan, T. Granneman, M. Harrigan, N. Holden, R. Phillips, J. Schore, C. Thornton, J. D. Wooldridge, and F. Skidmore, *The Evaluation of the National Long-term Care Demonstrations Final Report*, Mathematica Policy Research, Inc., Princeton, New Jersey, 1986.
11. R. Applebaum and J. Christianson, Using Case Management to Monitor Community-based Long-term Care, *QRB, 14*, pp. 227-231, 1988.
12. K. L. Braun, L. Goto, and A. Lenzer, Patient Age and Satisfaction with Home Care, *Home Health Care Services Quarterly, 8*, pp. 79-96, 1987.
13. K. B. Haskins, J. Capitman, F. Colligen, B. Degraaf, and C. Yordi, *Evaluation of Community Long-term Care Demonstration Projects: Extramural Report*, Health Care Financing Administration, Baltimore, 1987.
14. N. N. Eustis and L. R. Fischer, Relationships Between Home Care Clients and Their Workers: Implications for Quality of Care, *The Gerontologist, 31*:4, pp. 447-456, 1991.
15. M. Carlsson-Agren, S. Berg, and C. G. Wenestam, Daily Life of the Oldest Old, *Journal of Sociology and Social Welfare, 19*:2, pp. 109-124, 1992.
16. C. P. Sabatino, Client Rights Regulations and the Autonomy of Home-Care Consumers, *Generations, XIV*:Supplement, pp. 21-24, 1990.
17. National Citizens' Coalition for Nursing Home Reform, *A Consumer Perspective on Quality of Care: The Residents' Point of View*, Washington, D.C., 1985.
18. W. Lustbader, *Counting on Kindness: The Dilemmas of Dependency*, The Free Press, New York, 1991.
19. D. Berwick and M. Knapp, Theory and Practice for Measuring Health Care Quality, *Health Care Financing Review, 9*:Supplement, pp. 49-55, 1987.

# CHAPTER
# 10

# Someone To Come By:
# The Social Component of Formal Care

*Just to have people come by two or three days a week is a big help. When a person becomes disabled, people don't visit them often, even people you know well. Having them come by breaks the monotony. That's a help. I get a chance to talk to people.*

Rev. Joseph Scott

Rev. Scott cannot walk, but he is alert, informed, and naturally gregarious. He prepares and tape records spirited sermons for later broadcast on a local radio station. He continues to operate his small tax preparation business from his home. But, except for his aides, he often has no one to talk to. His visits from church members and family are only occasional, and, if he does not need Deacon Pate to take him to the clinic, he may not see another person for a week or two—at least one not being paid to visit him.

The social world of each of these seven African American elders has shrunk dramatically over the years as their physical abilities have diminished. No longer are they able to get out, go places, and mix with people as they once did; nor do they have as many friends or visitors. For some, this reduced social integration is aggravated by feelings of aloneness caused by the loss of friends and family members and their support. For the four individuals who live alone, these problems are especially troublesome. Formal caregivers may provide the only contact they have during a day or even a week. Geraldine Starr and Sally Finch, although residents of senior highrises, remain sequestered in their apartments. Mr. Avant offers Eloise Little meager company, despite sharing her home. Even Lucy Oliver, whose husband is always with her, craves diverse social contacts.

The meaning of social interaction with formal care workers varies for these older persons. It is defined differently and serves different roles. As Rev. Scott states, the contact in and of itself is a help. It breaks up the day and provides a means of conversation. For Viola Worth, contact with her aide, Anne, offers her companionship and pleasurable activity:

> I look forward to her. We have fun!

These social interactions are not always positive experiences. When describing a different aide, Rev. Scott's tribute was somewhat qualified:

> Sometimes you have some to come in with a nasty attitude. I always say they don't need the job. Like I was at one time—particularly sick, anxious to see somebody—some of the ladies wouldn't talk. Ought to try to spread a little sunshine. One lady, not a regular, said, "I don't have any male patients anymore. They all died." I would have asked for a change [if she had been his regular]. If I'm feeling sad and someone comes in here with a sad face, it doesn't do me any good.

Like many aspects of caregiving, the importance of the social component of care is idiosyncratic. The meaning of the social contacts and the impact they have on clients are influenced by the personal characteristics of the individuals involved, such as the personality of an aide, the condition and preferences of the client, and by what transpires during the interactions.

While these clients find conversation with aides enjoyable and often conducive to fostering friendships, how conversation is viewed and experienced is conditional. They have rules about appropriate times and subjects for conversation. Being alone with no one to talk to does *not* mean that just any conversation is welcome. When talk interferes with necessary tasks or makes a client unhappy or anxious, it is avoided. When it makes clients feel good or is rewarding in other ways, it is eagerly encouraged.

Moreover, close affective bonds tend to develop only when participants find such ties rewarding. When relationships with formal workers provide clients with friendship or family-like ties they value, clients view such relationships as beneficial and work to maintain them. Ms. Worth and Rev. Scott care more about developing such bonds than do Mrs. Washington, who has her husband and son close by, or Mrs. Finch, who is less sociable. On the other hand, if close affective bonds lead to controlling or other unwelcome interactions or if the aide has traits a client dislikes, clients look for ways to distance themselves from, or even to end, the relationship.

Aides use similar strategies to manage relationships in ways that are rewarding (or at least less burdensome) to them. When close ties are desired, they encourage clients' affection through the care they provide, and when emotional involvement is not attractive or too burdensome, restraint is maintained.

While the manifest functions of these formally provided home care services pertain primarily to basic physical care, most providers seem mindful of their clients' socio-emotional needs in the planning and delivery of services. Just having someone come into the home provides an additional social contact, and the social interchanges incumbent in the performance of routine physical caregiving duties affect (both positively and negatively) the socio-emotional state of the care receivers. A natural blending of the social and instrumental components of providing care occur during caregiving. In this chapter our focus is on social aspects of the formal caregiving experience as we examine more closely the nature of social interactions and interpersonal relationships between clients and their aides.

## SOMEONE TO TALK TO:
## THE IMPORTANCE OF CONVERSATION

*Sometimes when I'm here by myself a lot and don't have anyone to talk to, I think that I might forget how to communicate. I always enjoy talking to people.*

Rev. Joseph Scott

These clients have specific attitudes about the social conversation that goes on during an aide's visit—that is, whether they like conversation and what they like to talk about. Rev. Scott is a person who particularly enjoys talking to people and misses the frequent conversations he once had with former friends and parishioners. For him, visits from his aides afford opportunities for these missed conversations. Ms. Worth, too, treasures her chats with Anne:

You help me if we don't do nothing but sit down and talk.

Other authors describe similar experiences of clients with divergent ethnic and cultural backgrounds. Kate Quinton, the Irish-American client portrayed by Sheehan [1], enjoyed chatting, watching television, and sharing a glass of sherry with her aides. The older clients in Minnesota described by Eustis and Fischer [2] also valued the conversation and companionship of their formal care providers.

Be that as it may, we found clients to have rules about conversation—about when and how it should proceed and about its content. As noted in Chapter 9, as a rule, clients believe social conversation should not take priority over, or replace, the provision of basic physical care. Mrs. Little expressed this view when she complained about her aides talking instead of working:

> She [one aide] talks too much. She comes here to clean up. Well she don't do it—just sits down and talks.

Mrs. Little's comment does not mean she dislikes talking to her aide. It simply means she *also* likes her aide to perform needed chores:

> She's real nice. She do a little work and sit down and talk. I likes that.

Rev. Scott enjoys conversing with his home health aide *while* she works and would prefer longer dialogues, but these conversations do not take precedence over basic care:

> She's a good talker. We talk while she works. She does what she's supposed to do while she's here. She doesn't spend any time around after she finishes up. Sometimes they do have a heavy schedule, have to rush off to the next one.

And Ms. Worth is unwilling to give up her bath:

> I just enjoy Anne. I don't care if she don't do nothing but help me with my bath, and we sit here and talk.

Here too the issue of client control is key. As Ms. Worth notes below, it is sometimes permissible, even preferred, to talk rather than work—when it is the *client's* decision:

> Anne doesn't sit around and talk. If we *want* to sit and rap, we do.

The client then must determine the appropriateness of "sitting and talking."

Some of these clients, however, do not place as much value on social conversation, nor do clients always feel like talking. Mrs. Finch, for

one, prefers that her aide leave as soon as she has completed the
necessary tasks:

> No need in two hours [the allotted time for the visit], if just sittin'
> there talking all the time. Give me a bath and go. Don't sit around
> and talk.

As noted earlier, Mrs. Finch tends to get nervous in groups and prefers
to keep to herself. Mrs. Starr at times also finds conversation with
aides annoying:

> I get tired of talking too. You [the aide] come in that door talking,
> and I don't even *feel* like talking.

These varying, and sometimes contradictory, client preferences
emphasize the ambiguity of the home care aide's role. Eustis and
Fischer noted the difficulty some aides had in defining the parameters
of their responsibilities [2]. One case in point involved a client's
daughter who wanted the aide to put more emphasis on housekeeping
chores while the mother preferred the aide watch TV and play cards
with her.

We found these clients have additional dictums about the manner in
which conversation should proceed and appropriate topics for conversation. One rule concerns the asking of questions, which at times is
viewed as inappropriate and, by some, downright aggravating. Mrs.
Starr is particularly perturbed by being questioned. Behavior that her
aide, Myrtice, defines as, "just concerned," to Mrs. Starr is "nosy":

> I'm kind of glad Myrtice ain't here. She aggravated the hell out of
> me. She's a big talker, too. She just asked a whole bunch of ques-
> tions. Nosy, nosy rosy. I don't like nosy people. She asked a lot of
> unnecessary things, audacious questions. Let *me* tell you if I want
> you to know. I want somebody to tell *me* something.

While Mrs. Starr finds these questions irksome, they also represent an
invasion of privacy. Refusing to answer is a strategy she uses to control
information, a way to retain power or independence in the relationship—that is, the less one knows about me, the more independent I am.
Mrs. Starr wants to make the decision about what personal facts to
divulge, and she flatly refuses to answer what seems like a trivial
question—the identity of an individual in a photograph on her dresser.
Mrs. Starr's preference would be for the aide to give *her* information,
information that she might use to improve her situation. In other

conversations she has let it be known that she likes to learn, particularly about her condition and about general health care.

Irritability about answering questions also stems from the fact that these clients receive services from a variety of bureaucratic institutions and routinely face interrogations. Typically, the same questions are asked repeatedly, and many questions are quite personal or seem inconsequential. It is not surprising that offense is taken at "unnecessary" questions. This same attitude sometimes made probing for information a touch-and-go affair, as evidenced by the first author's experience when she asked Mrs. Starr what she meant by "audacious questions," only to receive the reply, "Now, there *you* go." A more successful strategy proved to be commenting nonchalantly on the subject of interest and let the information flow.

The topic of conversation is a critical element in whether these clients welcome discourse with their aides. Mrs. Finch expresses the commonly held view that conversation should be about happy or pleasant topics:

> But you know what? People mostly having troubles. Tell you their troubles, especially with the children. I like to talk about things that happened long time ago, something to laugh about. There's too much sadness.

Already depressed about her own situation, she prefers more cheerful exchanges. Mrs. Starr, also regularly dispirited, related how an aide's tale about the robbery of an old woman upset her:

> I *got* something to worry about—walking again. It went all over me.

Eustis and Fischer found that the home care aides they studied were aware of similar client attitudes, and they were cautious about sharing personal information that might trouble their clients [2].

Compatibility in age, interests, or worldview can influence clients' attitudes toward the value of social conversation. Rev. Scott avoids conversation about what he considers "immoral behavior:"

> Well, I realize they come here for a purpose, to do a certain amount of work, but I wouldn't want somebody coming in that drinks. Like one time I had somebody coming in and the whole conversation was about the down side of life and about the kind of night life she was involved in on weekends. Well, I'm not interested in such as that.

Being a minister, he prefers an aide who shares, or at least respects, his values and views. The topic of conversation this particular aide chose was offensive to him. Sheehan described a similar incident when an aide's vulgar language upset a client [1].

Mrs. Finch enjoys talking about old times and has difficulty conversing with younger aides:

> Oh yeah, I don't mind talking to Elizabeth [her HMA]. She's older. Just like these little young girls. I don't know what to say to 'em. If I be trying to tell 'em something, they ain't gonna listen no way. Ain't no need in me talking. I can't talk to young people. They don't know.

In one situation, racial differences created a barrier to conversation. With the exception of Anne, Ms. Worth's PCA, the aides that visit these seven clients are also African American. Ms. Worth loves Anne and is not bothered by her being white. When Anne became Rev. Scott's aide, however, he found the racial disparity more problematic:

> Well, it's kind of a new experience. Only once before I had a white nurse [aide] come from VNA, and that was because someone was out. It was only for two weeks. Anne seems real nice. It's all right. I just feel more comfortable with somebody else. I always thought of whites as being supervisors and trainers rather than being regular aides. If that's the way it have to be, I'll go along with it. It's just somebody of my race would have more to talk about, things that are happening in the neighborhood as such.

Rev. Scott's discomfort with having a white aide was related to a perceived incompatibility, as well as to the lack of fit with his expectations for the typical role of white home care personnel. In Ms. Worth's case, she and Anne share the experience of being a woman, and her experiences and relationships with white people have been generally positive. She lived for many years in the homes of her employers, whom she described with affection, often minimizing their racial differences. Her feelings about having a white aide were clear:

> I *love* it! I come up [was raised] with white people. I don't have . . . I can't say that big word [prejudice]. I don't have stuff like that. No, don't mess with my Anne now. I'm just me. You [the researcher] treat me right. I know that you're white and I'm black, but we all human. The white people have taken up for me when the blacks haven't, but I love any of 'em that treat me right. Talking about color, baby—only thing, you treat me right, and we try to get along with one another. That color ain't gonna pay nairy bills. That color ain't gonna put nothing in my stomach. Be nice and everything will

work out. If we had more of that, the world would be a better place. But getting back to my girl [Anne], Allen [a neighbor] mentioned one day, "Miss Viola got a white lady." I say, that lady got to make a living just like I have. I say, don't worry about the color. I say, she is out there to make a living just like I was. I'm crazy about my Anne.

With Rev. Scott, Anne was only a temporary aide, but since she demonstrates in her care of Ms. Worth many of the traits Rev. Scott admires—for example, competence and a caring and willing attitude—it is likely, had she remained with him, his discomfort would have diminished.

## SOME JUST GET CLOSER: THE NATURE OF RELATIONSHIPS

*I ain't got nobody. She means a lot to me. My life has been a lots better. I'm not quite as crabby as I was, not as angry. She cuts it off. She's really good for my ego, good for my everything. I wouldn't want nobody better than her. She's so sweet. She makes it like I got somebody.*

Geraldine Starr

Sometimes close interpersonal relationships develop between clients and aides. In some cases these relationships help fulfill clients' needs for the socio-emotional bonds missing from their lives. In the passage quoted above, Mrs. Starr is referring to Lois, her senior companion, who during her tenure with Mrs. Starr assumed a primary caregiving role. The feeling Mrs. Starr got from Lois's care—like she "got somebody"—came not only from the extent of physical care that Lois provided, but also from the affection and friendship she offered. Lois made a difference in many aspects of Mrs. Starr's life as a dependent person, and a substantial part of that difference derived from the social component of care. We found these close relationships between clients and their aides often take on characteristics more typical of ties between family and friends.

### Aides As Family

Ms. Worth has developed close ties with past aides and now has come to view her present aide, Anne, "like family":

That girl is a mess. She put me in the mind of one I used to have. She come to be just part of me. She would pick up stuff to help me with my appetite, got me started to eating again, looked out for me [tried to find] a vacuum cleaner, got my garbage can on sale. That girl was just like family. Anne is the same way. She is going to look for me a cap when she goes shopping. That make you feel good. We just done got close. I just hope they don't take my Anne.

"Claiming family" is a strategy Ms. Worth uses to increase her informal caregiving network, and here she claims Anne as family to cement their relationship. This strategy is used only when formal workers exhibit the necessary traits, and not all do:

Some are more gentler than others, just their nature. Some of 'em we just get closer, more like family than others. Everybody's got their way of doing.

Anne is sweet and kind, and she goes out of her way to help Ms. Worth, even leaving her real family on Christmas day to bring dinner. Ms. Worth has "claimed" Anne's son as her grandson, and she and Anne confide in each other about their families and other personal matters. This behavior fits Ms. Worth's definition of family, a relationship she values, and she happily incorporates Anne into her "homemade family."

Like Ms. Worth, Mrs. Starr is estranged from her sons and has few other consanguinal kin ties. Since Lois left, she has become close to her aide, Vicky, whom she views in some ways as a daughter. They often talk about Vicky's own family, and Vicky has brought her two daughters to visit on the weekends. Vicky does not go out of her way to be helpful in the way that Anne does for Ms. Worth, nor does she perform her caregiving tasks as thoroughly or competently. Yet, Vicky understands Mrs. Starr's ways, and she has a quiet manner about her that pleases Mrs. Starr and gives her support:

Vicky came and stayed awhile. See, I feel strong when somebody's around me. That's something new to me. I'm used to being by myself.

Mrs. Starr allows herself to feel an affection for Vicky she will not concede to her highrise neighbors, who she believes have nothing to offer her.

## Aides As Friends

Rev. Scott frequently laments the loss of friends that has accompanied his disability and subsequent dependency. In discussions of relationships with informal caregivers, he names only Deacon Pate as a friend, but he counts two of his aides among his friends. He defines them as friends because of their social roles and because of the kind of basic care they provide. In the following passage, he explains his friendship with his homemaker aide, Mrs. Conner:

> Well, I think she would be classed as a friend because what she does is try to be helpful. I know she has certain guidelines to follow, certain things that she is supposed to do when she comes, but, in addition to that, I think she's a friend. We talk a lot of times while she's working. She seems to be a nice person. She said on one occasion, she didn't want to take anything from me, she'd rather give me something. Sometimes when she's working, if she doesn't have to rush off to another job, she'll do a few little extra things, take a little extra time.

Rev. Scott's criteria for friendship include Mrs. Conner's willingness to be helpful beyond her required role, her commitment to give, rather than take, and their conversations.

He also defines his home health aide, Mrs. Ellis, as a friend:

> Well, Mrs. Ellis, she's a type of a friend. We talk. She did call while I was in the hospital to see how I was getting along, although she didn't come to see me. When I got back home, she called to see if I was here.

As noted earlier, Mrs. Ellis's schedule does not allow her time to sit and talk after finishing her work. Still, they converse while she works, and she has made the extra effort to check on him in the hospital. This behavior justifies Rev. Scott's label of her as friend.

Mrs. Finch's homemaker aide, Elizabeth, has some of the same traits that fit Rev. Scott's criteria for friendship—enjoyable conversation, being helpful, and taking extra time. Yet, because Mrs. Finch defines friendship differently, Elizabeth is not a friend:

> She doin' what she supposed to do. Anybody that don't visit [on a social basis], I wouldn't consider them as my friend.

Elizabeth's visits are in the line of duty, not social visits, which, for Mrs. Finch, are necessary acts of friendship.

For Rev. Scott, a formal worker can be viewed as both a professional and a friend. In fact, because of past experiences with former aides, he insists that these relationships remain professional—making a conscious effort not to become personally involved, keeping interactions restricted to official visits, and referring to them by their last names. He described how this attitude developed:

> Well, people feel free to talk about their personal problems, seek a little advice. I remember saying to someone once that we should keep our relationship professional, talking when here but not get involved in their problems in a way that would be harmful as such. I may have told you about a lady that got fired—we kind of got to know one another just talking and going on, and she got to the point where she felt she could borrow money from me, and I let her have it, and she got to the point where she didn't want to pay it back. I had to let the company know about it and asked for a wage assignment on it. I never did get the money back. They just fired her. I found out she was doing some other people the same way. Well, it helped me in a way that I knew not to let them have money again. . . . When this [another experience] happened she was talking about her personal problems. Her husband didn't get paid off. She brought her children over here after dark one night, said she didn't have any food. I didn't have any money for her. I felt kind of sorry for her, and I let her have a little food out of my Frigerdare, enough to take care of a few days. The little children thanked me for it. I guess I just felt for them. I felt that she could ask me. That was getting involved. The experience I had with her let me know not to get too involved.

Rev. Scott now keeps sufficient personal distance between himself and his aides to prevent future exploitive situations, but not too great a distance to impede the development of friendships. Whereas social relationships are often shunned by Mrs. Finch, friendship is highly valued by Rev. Scott, and he actively tries to make friends:

> I try to conduct myself in such a way that I could have friends. There is a saying that, "He who would have friends, must *be* a friend," and I try to be a friend, hoping that I could have some good friends.

Even though his aide might not conform to the typical definition of a friend, Rev. Scott has redefined the situation to fit his values. Rosenberg has designated this "selectivity of values," a strategy to enhance self-esteem [3]. Rev. Scott defines the relationship as one of friendship because having friends is important to him and he has few other alternatives to satisfy this need. Other studies of friendships in late life also reported that older people commonly revise their criteria for friendship, at times expanding the definition to include paid help [4, 5].

A critical element in the development of close affective bonds is whether aides perform their duties in ways that demonstrate to clients their care and concern for them as human beings. As discussed in the preceding chapter, this understanding can develop even when aides perform only routine caregiving tasks, but some aides find extra ways of showing they care. As one aide explained:

> That's the kind of thing [the first author had brought an Easter basket] I like to do, fix stuff like that, valentines. My patients [are] like my kids. I get a big charge out of all my patients. I got one that really drives me crazy, but I really look forward to seeing that lady, and if I go and she's not home, then I'm worried to death about her, and I will call till she gets home.

It is clear that a certain type of aide makes a special effort to provide socio-emotional support as an integral part of their caregiving. As Ms. Worth said, it's "their nature." Eustis and Fischer found two-thirds of the clients they studied reported their workers provided extra services, beyond their scheduled time and duties, and the authors associated this expansion of the normal job boundaries with the development of personal ties between clients and their workers [2]. In this study, almost two-thirds of clients and about half of the aides defined their relationships as friend- or family-like.

Other aides, however, have traits that cause clients to resist close relationships, such as an aide Rev. Scott described:

> Well it depends on the kind of treatment they give. This lady from another agency, when she first started coming, she was a nervous-acting person, like she's afraid to come here, afraid of men, like she might have thought every man comes around might have wanted her or something like that. Some food she cooked for me I ate, I got that feeling like I had when I was taking salt tablets. I couldn't prove that she had put something like that in my food, but I had heard of people trying to control patients as such. Sometimes when they kind of get to know you they change a little bit, but you don't always know.

In this case, Rev. Scott was not comfortable being with the aide and did not trust her, and it is unlikely that an effort would be made by either to develop a close relationship.

In some situations, workers remain with clients for extended periods of time, even up to two years. Such was the case with the two aides Rev. Scott considered his friends and Mrs. Finch's homemaker aide, Elizabeth. Although a lengthy relationship was not always necessary for close affective bonds to develop—Ms. Worth, for example, "got close" to Anne soon after she became her aide—these participants' relationships with their aides generally did not continue, at least to any significant extent, after the official aide/client relationship ended. Anne was transferred from Ms. Worth to another client shortly after the research period ended, and in the ensuing six months, Ms. Worth spoke with her only once by telephone. But Ms. Worth has no regrets about this relationship, only fond memories of both Anne and Caroline, the other aide to whom she was close:

> I wouldn't ever forget her [Anne]. I still love her. She's right next to Caroline.

Like the clients described by Eustis and Fischer [2], these clients would prefer to keep aides they have become fond of, but they are pragmatic about the situation, understanding that it is an area over which they have little control. Though they know they can never count on the long-term availability of their aides, those clients who have developed close affective ties believe the benefits of a close relationship usually outweigh the costs.

Aides, too, feel close to clients, but considering their heavy workloads and the more pressing needs of ongoing clients, maintaining relationships with former clients can be cumbersome. One aide described how she managed to keep up with a former client who needed her support:

> I don't do her anymore, but on my easy days I stop by and see her, and I call her and see how she's doing. She don't have any family, and sometimes on the weekends, if she need something, I'll drive all the way back out here to go to the store for her.

Because of possible emotional costs, some aides actively resist getting too close to clients. One aide, who was with Mrs. Oliver only a short time, explained how she severs relationships that are potentially too hurtful:

> It's good to love 'em and take good care of 'em, but when you get so attached and something happens, it's awful. It's awful when they die. Just be so sad. So when I start getting too attached, I move out.

Costs also occur for clients when close ties exist. When Rev. Scott became too personally involved with his aide and loaned her money, the experience for him was both emotionally and financially expensive. In Mrs. Starr's situation, being close to Vicky makes it harder for her to direct Vicky in the basic caregiving tasks, a role that Mrs. Starr already finds difficult. As we shall see in Chapter 11, her close relationship with Vicky sometimes interferes with the process of care. She admits the problematic nature of their relationship:

> I done ruined her. She plays with me and hugs me.

The following excerpts from their conversation give further evidence:

| | |
|---|---|
| Mrs. Starr: | Don't come in here trying to fall down. You ain't able to stand up. Just come on in here and sit down. |
| Vicky: | I'm gonna eat and run. |
| Mrs. Starr: | That's all you do. I'm going to report all of you. You and Peggy [another aide] both. |
| Vicky: | Maybe they'll fire me and I can rest. |
| Mrs. Starr: | I don't want you fired. I want you to stay on. Where have you been all day? |
| Vicky: | I've been to Buckhead, Bankhead Highway, and I got to go elsewhere and then home. |
| Mrs. Starr: | Where the devil is elsewhere? If I keep fooling with Vicky, I'm going loco, nutty too. I worry to death about her. . . . I see your thighs. Where's your husband? Don't walk around here showing your meat. |
| Vicky: | I know the trash needs taking out, what else you want me to do? |
| Mrs. Starr: | What I need for today? Money. |
| Vicky: | I say what you need me to *do*? |
| Mrs. Starr: | Stay here and look at me, and I look at you. I'll hold on to my baby. That's my baby. Tell her she better not go out that door. I ain't ready to let you go. |

In the above interaction, Mrs. Starr is more focused on the social aspect of their relationship than on what caregiving tasks Vicky might accomplish. During that particular visit of two hours, she only swept the floor and emptied the trash, spending the remainder of her time eating her lunch and talking to Mrs. Starr.

As noted in Chapter 9, problems also developed in Mrs. Starr's relationship with Lois. As Lois became more involved in all aspects of her client's care, she began to assume more control, even taking on a managerial role. Despite Mrs. Starr's affection for Lois and the instrumental and emotional support Lois provided, at a certain point Mrs. Starr could tolerate no longer the extent of Lois's caregiving role. Eustis and Fischer found similar tensions between personal and professional role relationships [2]. Workers felt exploited by informal arrangements without clearcut boundaries around work expectations, finding it particularly difficult to be treated as "just workers" by clients who were also friends. Clients, on the other hand, felt deserted by former aides and friends who no longer visited them. Sheehan described an especially caring aide who ultimately had to leave her client and the home care profession because of the unreasonably high demands on her time that resulted from close interpersonal ties with the client [1]. Another of her clients became resentful and resistent to care when her independence, like that of Mrs. Starr, was threatened by the aide's competent care.

* * * * *

For the seven clients participating in this study, the social component of the formal home care services is most important for those who live alone and for those who most value social interactions as a part of their everyday life. Conversation is happily engaged in, as long as certain rules are followed. Close affective bonds—even family-like ties—develop when both aides and clients have the traits that encourage development and when opportunities exist for both their development and their continuation. A key determinant of the value for the care receiver of the more social aspects of the caregiving experience is again the caregiver's willingness to provide care according to the client's choices and directions.

In the next chapter we will examine the client's own role in the caregiving process. The personal relationship between the client and the aide is just one factor that influences a client's particular role definition.

# REFERENCES

1. S. Sheehan, *Kate Quinton's Days,* New American Library, New York, 1984.
2. N. N. Eustis and L. R. Fischer, Relationships Between Home Care Clients and Their Workers: Implications for Quality of Care, *The Gerontologist, 31*:4, pp. 447-456, 1991.
3. M. Rosenberg, *Conceiving the Self,* Basic Books, New York, 1979.
4. C. L. Johnson and L. E. Troll, Constraints and Facilitators to Friendships in Late Late Life, *The Gerontologist, 34*:1, pp. 79-87, 1994.
5. B. M. Barer, The Relationship Between Homebound Older People and Their Home Care Worker, *Journal of Gerontological Social Work, 19*, pp. 129-147, 1992.

# CHAPTER
# 11

# Making the Client Role

*I haven't bothered her about cooking. I'd just rather do for myself. . . . Yeah, she'll fix me something to eat if I want her to, but I keep trying to do something for myself, like my mind tells me to do.*

Geraldine Starr

For Geraldine Starr, mornings are her "hardest time." She wakes up tired. Most days her bed and night clothes are wet from urine. She has to wash herself right away to keep her skin from chafing, and she likes to gather the urine-soaked bed clothes so her aide will not have to touch them. Several of her medications are to be taken early and with food, but she feels too weak to prepare break-fast when she first arises. If Vicky came earlier, she could help, but Mrs. Starr has been unable to schedule her homemaker services in the morning. By the time mid-afternoon rolls around and Vicky does arrive, Mrs. Starr has gained a little energy and chooses to do her own cooking.

The very nature of social welfare policies often encourages continu-ing dependency [1]. Clients' acceptance of the dependent state in fact can reduce conflict in provider-client interactions and facilitate the task of providing care [2]. At the same time, providers are frequently frustrated by what they consider unnecessary client dependencies or their unwillingness to perform tasks they are capable of doing [1].

We found, however, that these African American clients in most instances try to avoid dependency. Instead, they cling to the vestiges of their independence while enacting their client roles. This attitude toward self-reliance is just one of the factors that influence their behaviors as clients. It is clear that the actions clients choose—how they define and act out their roles in the formal caregiving process—affect significantly the outcomes of their formal caregiving experiences. In this chapter we show how these participants develop

205

and define their roles as clients and how their personal role definitions influence the caregiving process and the quality of care.

## MAKING ROLES

Roles define how individuals holding a particular position in society are expected to behave. These roles carry with them specific expectations for behavior that persist independently of the person occupying the position. Within the interactionist framework, roles exist in varying degrees of concreteness and consistency, providing only a general framework for behavior [3]. Role incumbents not only "take" (assume) roles but create and modify ("make") them. Even in the most rigidly defined situation, the creative processes associated with role-taking and role-making are in constant operation. The extent to which roles are individually molded or "made," rather than simply "played," depends on the larger social structures in which the interactive situations are embedded [4]. All structures impose some limitations on how roles are defined and the latitude actors have to make modifications.

Because a role exists only in relation to other roles, interaction is always a tentative process. Actors are continuously devising their performances based on their conceptions of the imputed other-role [5]. The sources of behavioral expectations may be from society at large, from people enacting the same and reciprocal roles, and from the self [6].

Thornton and Nardi describe a developmental approach to role acquisition that emphasizes the process of adjustment to roles and the interaction between individuals and their roles [6]. Their model sets forth four stages of role acquisition: anticipatory, formal, informal, and personal. These four stages do not have equal importance for all roles, but complete adaptation to a role requires enactment of all four stages. Each stage is defined by the types of expectation that predominate and involves interactions between role incumbents and external expectations. Individuals enacting roles and their partners both attempt to influence the other, with role behavior typically becoming more active with the progression of stages.

In the anticipatory stage, people develop preconceptions about new roles primarily from generalized sources and from others occupying similar roles. Once individuals enter the anticipated role, expectations are formalized and arise typically from members of the same role set. When roles are part of organizational structures, expectations tend to be explicitly written, listed, and stated. In other, more loosely defined situations, few formal expectations are present. Thornton and Nardi suggest that initial success in role acquisition is partly dependent on the closeness of fit between these first two stages [6].

The informal stage involves unofficial expectations that are implicit, rather than explicit, and are transmitted through interactions with individuals. Personal expectations become more important at this stage, and individuals begin to shape their roles and formulate their own meanings for performance.

In the personal stage, role acquisition includes a psychological dimension, which allows individuals' unique personalities to come into play. It is at this stage, Thornton and Nardi suggest, that individuals impose their own style on role performance, critical for social and psychological adjustment and for full adaptation to a role [6]. Without this molding of self to role, enactment tends to be perfunctory and performance ineffective.

## MAKING THE CLIENT ROLE

Although the role of the home care client is an officially recognized component of the formal caregiving system, most regulations that concern clients pertain to eligibility requirements relating to finances and to health status. Few formal directives exist to specify how client roles should be enacted. Rights and duties are loosely defined rather than rigidly prescribed, allowing clients considerable latitude to develop uniquely defined roles. The fact that role performance routinely takes place within the client's home creates additional opportunities for molding client roles to individual situations and needs. Home care providers, however, have certain implicit, if not explicit, expectations for the client role. Clients should believe they need the services provided, should furnish accurate information, should strive for the highest level of independence, and should not maximize or minimize their problems [7]. It is safe to say the providers serving our informants generally share these expectations. Additionally, they expect clients, or their informal caregivers, will know what services they are authorized to receive and who is providing them, will communicate their service needs to their home care aides, and will report service problems to the appropriate supervisor. Such information about services and procedures is regularly communicated to clients by the various service providers, particularly the case managers and RN supervisors. Clients, however, do not always hear and assimilate the information appropriately, nor do they always act in the expected manner.

Each of these older persons has been receiving formal home care services for a number of years. Already familiar with the client role, they have progressed through what Thornton and Nardi refer to as the anticipatory and formal stages of role acquisition [6]. While they regularly encounter more formalized expectations (for example, during annual assessments or periodic case reviews), these are not rigidly defined or explicit prescriptions for behavior. It is in the final two stages, the informal and the personal, that clients formulate their own meanings for the client role and individually mold its performance. It is at this point that expectations of the members of clients' role sets—primarily the aides but also those in supervisory positions—and those of the clients themselves exert their influences.

Within the structural limitations of the formal caregiving system, these clients have created personalized client roles. Each role is an expression of the client's quest for attainment of specific goals related to their unique caregiving needs. Each role has been molded in response to expectations developed during ongoing interactions of clients and caregivers and to expectations clients have developed for themselves based on their personal attitudes, values, skills, and abilities. While clients vary in the degree they modify or "make" these roles to suit their own needs and in the extent they fully adapt to the client role, it is clear they are not just passive recipients of their services. Care is not always just done *to* them and *for* them. Rather, to the extent that their resources permit, these participants take an active role in both the content and process of care. These roles are creative adaptations to each client's own particular circumstances, and, as such, they are *made* rather than only *played*.

In-home care clients generally interact with two levels of formal workers—those who directly provide the services—in this study aides and RN's—and those in supervisory positions—case managers and RN's, who sometimes also provide care. By examining the behavior of these seven clients in and around their interactions with these two levels of workers, we will show how the client role develops, focusing on the factors molding its development and the consequences of its ultimate definition. While not adhering strictly to the Thornton and Nardi [6] model, we will use its major concepts as a guide in analyzing how these older, impaired persons create their roles as clients.

## GETTING HELP FROM AIDES

With these seven clients, it is in their interactions with their aides that the most profound shaping of the client role takes place. As the preceding chapters make clear, aides vary a great deal in how they deliver care. Clients differ as well in how they wish care to be provided.

The successes these clients have in getting adequate care often hinges on the success of their personal strategies.

## Asking for Help

A critical component of the client role is whether clients ask their aides for the help they need. Direct, verbal communications between clients and caregivers involve making requests for particular services and giving instructions about how they wish tasks to be performed. While program regulations specify which tasks aides are authorized to provide, and clients have care plans based on their unique needs, sometimes plans are abandoned, and sometimes the authorized tasks are not what clients want or believe they need. We found that despite service deficiencies, clients often do not ask for help, and their failure to communicate their needs can have significant impacts on the process of care.

Three kinds of factors influence whether clients ask aides for help—those that relate to their beliefs and values, those dependent on particular knowledge or abilities, and those associated with client-aide bonds. Clients' attitudes toward their independence and control, the work of aides, and the rights and responsibilities of the client role are key factors affecting their behavior. Another dimension comes from their abilities to understand the home care program, evaluate their own needs for care, and make these needs known to aides. The nature of the interactive process itself further influences the client role—how aides respond to clients' requests and the dynamics of client-caregiver encounters. To ask for help clients must have the physical and mental abilities and the supportive beliefs and values that allow them to identify needs, organize and plan needed care, be motivated to ask for help, know whom to ask, make the request, and be willing to accept the help. They also must perceive caregivers as not only able but willing to provide the necessary care. The presence of the right combination of resources and attitudes of both caregivers and care receivers is necessary for client action.

### Client Attitudes

*Independence Revisited.* Each of these clients holds a strong value for independence and usually, when able, will choose to perform a task independently. As in interactions with informal caregivers, this value influences whether clients ask their aides for help and often restricts the role of formal caregivers. Because of her proclivity for self-reliance, Sally Finch typically limits the activities of her aides:

> She supposed to help with my bath. Most of the time I be done straightened up the bed. If I have dishes in the sink, she'll do that. She'll ask, "You want me to fix you something?" Most of the time I be done et my toast and coffee. They would cook, but I'd rather do it myself, as long as I'm able. They're supposed to make your beds and things if you can't do it yourself, but I do it myself. There a heap of things they supposed to do, I do myself. I ask Martha [the HA] to do the things I can't do. I don't want to ask some things. Ain't no need in just sittin' here when I feel like it. As long as able, you ought to try to help yourself. I try to do the best I can. If I don't do nothing, it's bad, if you just sit in one place and don't do nothing. Some people don't do nothing.

A client's independent behavior sometimes is reinforced by an aide's unsatisfactory job performance. While Mrs. Starr frequently pleads for more help (particularly in the area of cooking), her dissatisfaction with Vicky's efforts bolsters her determination to continue "doin' for herself":

> I can go in that bathroom and sit in that chair and wash things. I don't do too much rubbing because I don't get my things dirty. Vicky don't have time to rinse 'em good, so I just fix them myself. As long as I feel, I mean I got a little strength, I'm gonna use it. No point in just holding up. . . . Vicky plaits my hair too tight. I told her to do it looser, but she got such a hand, so I do for myself as long as I can.

And Mrs. Finch's penchant to cook for herself is fortified by her past displeasure with her aide's culinary practices:

> I don't bother my nurses. She put the bacon in the pot and got on the telephone. I never asked no more. I don't like fast cooking.

*Client Control.* Clients may be daunted in their quests for help by beliefs that aides are reluctant to perform the services they request. Because they experience in these interactions many of the same emotions that cloud their relationships with informal caregivers, these old people often feel powerless to influence the behavior of their aides. Bloom and Wilson suggest that experts in any delivery of services have certain initiatives that afford power and create asymmetry in relationships [8]. This asymmetry, they note, can create formidable barriers to communication and mutual satisfaction. Such barriers influence the relationships of these clients with their physicians, and parallels exist in their formal home care experiences. When deemed an expert in some aspect of home care, an RN, or even a home health care aide, becomes more powerful in the client's estimation.

The client's perceived impotence often is substantiated during caregiving interactions. When aides display less-than-willing attitudes, as Rev. Scott describes in the passage below, clients are loath to request a desired service:

> Yes, but they might not want to do what you ask sometimes, but you can tell 'em what you want, and if they don't want to do it, they'll show it in some way. If they don't show it, they might act it out. I had one lady coming, she was to do some cooking one day. I asked if she could make a meatloaf. She made the meatloaf, but I couldn't eat it. I wondered if that was her way of saying, "Don't ask me to cook any more." I sure didn't.

When past requests have been disregarded, clients are reluctant to ask again, as Mrs. Starr explains:

> I told her about the floor, and she said she would mop up, but she didn't. I tell 'em but they just don't do it. Joanne won't do nothing no more. I don't know what to tell her to do because she does just the opposite. She just wants to walk out the door. What good does it do me to tell 'em if they don't do it, half do, or do just the opposite. I just lay here and watch.

Even a client like Ms. Worth, who is more keen on, and adept at, making requests, can be discouraged from future appeals by aides' recalcitrance:

> I got to where I didn't want to ask her to do nothing because she doesn't half do. I talked to her, "If you just do one room, just do it right." I tried to give her a chance. I said it to her.

As with informal caregivers, feelings of powerlessness can elicit more passive strategies to retain control—doing without the needed service.

On the other hand, a willing aide with an obliging attitude stimulates clients to take the more active tack, as Ms. Worth does with her current aide, Anne:

> Anne do things. I got a job for her when she come here Wednesday. I got to have some medicine. My aide can pick them up. She's

supposed to do things like that. Anne good. She'll do anything I ask.
I feel like if I didn't have anyone to do 'em [pay her bills], I think
she'd pay 'em for me. I believe she would.

It is through interactions with their aides during the process of
care that these clients develop certain attitudes about the efficacy of
their actions and assume the role behavior they believe is expected, if
only implicitly, by the caregiver. How caregivers present themselves to
care receivers—that is, willing or unwilling—and how they perform
their caregiving tasks influence whether clients actively seek their
help.

*Aides' Work.* The employment conditions for aides have been
described as deplorable. Their job is the least-skilled and lowest paid in
the home care industry; the hours are long and the work often is
unpleasant and frustrating [9, 10]. In some cases, empathetic clients
are less willing to ask workers to carry out certain tasks and more
disposed toward self-care.

Both Mrs. Starr and Ms. Worth empathize with their aides because
of the difficult aspects of home care work. These feelings are
intensified by memories of their personal work experiences. Mrs. Starr
explains how her identification with Vicky's role influences her own
behavior:

I didn't want to worry her. She's beat out. She's got a lot of bed
patients. Vicky has more than she can tend to. When she comes,
she's so tired. She ain't able to do for me. She can't do it. She just
comes and sits down. I don't say anything to her. Putting so many
people on the nurses will soon break 'em down, a leg-killin' job. I
wouldn't take that [that kind of work]. That's the reason I don't
have no Social Security.

Mrs. Starr's empathy is intensified by memories of caring for
her bedridden mother. Her attitudes toward taking care of her
mother's toileting needs color her view of her aide's personal care
duties. She still finds these chores distasteful, and she tries to spare
her aide:

I get up and wrap my Dependens [Depends—disposable
diapers] up. All she [the aide] has to do is pick it up. I know
I wouldn't want to put my hands on it. I tell her to get some gloves.
I don't want to put my hands on my own pee. I don't want to smell
'em.

Empathy develops also from listening to aides talk about their work. Ms. Worth's aide, Anne, confirmed the difficult and unpleasant aspects of her job:

> They [aides] start because it sounds great because there's nobody over your shoulder all the time, but then when you get out there, it's not what they expect because it's dirty diapers on some people, and you get someone that can't move, and it's a lot of strain. You have to care, too. When you give five baths a day, clean five houses, and you go home and you have to bathe your child and clean your house, it gets to you some days.

*Rights and Responsibilities.* Clients learn about the rights and responsibilities of the home care client role from other client-provider experiences (both past and present), from formal indoctrination to the client role, and from ongoing interactions during the process of care. Whether they believe they have both the right and the responsibility to ask for help and give instructions often determines the actions they take.

Ms. Worth's beliefs support a more assertive role. Her aide, Anne, endorses her behavior with encouraging words:

> The first visit is pretty much spent getting to know that patient. I want to discuss it—how you want your bed made. Ms. Worth has a certain way she wants her bed made. She had to show me. I don't want to do it and then leave and have her say she didn't do that like I wanted. I really want to know what that person wants.

Mrs. Starr, on the other hand, avoids this component of the client role. She believes that telling workers how to do their jobs is *not* her responsibility as a client. Nobody had to tell her when she was working, and, therefore, such direction should not be required of her:

> I don't tell 'em to do nothing. Listen, you're cleaning, you keeps your house, you go in somebody else's house, you do just like they do—see the paper, pick the paper up, see the stove dirty, just go ahead and clean it. I ain't got time. If they try to get by with it, that's they business. They supposed to check, and clean if not. Don't put it on me. I can't tell 'em what to do. Why they want to fault me? When I went somewhere to clean, I *knew* what to do. I don't need to tell somebody what to do. *They* got a house. White people didn't want to have to tell me. They'll put the blame on me, don't see anything to be done. They supposed to know.

Her feeling that Vicky should not have to endure the close monitoring she once tolerated gives her further cause to shirk the supervisory role:

> When I worked, the white ladies were all the time runnin' their hands over the furniture. I want you to do things the way you want. I don't want nobody watchin' over you.

Mrs. Starr's preference is to forfeit the rights and responsibilities she finds inappropriate and burdensome and give her aides freedom to go about their work as they choose.

Research that has investigated the aide's perspective suggests that Mrs. Starr's empathy is well-placed. Eustis and co-workers affirmed the negative impact of powerlessness on the well-being of home-care aides [11], and Surpin and Grumm found that aides struggle to avoid being treated as maids [12]. On the other hand, Stoller and Cutler reported that directing home care workers was less problematic for more affluent clients, for whom reliance on paid help was a way of life [13].

### Client Abilities

Certain knowledge and skills are essential for clients to ask for needed help. These abilities are closely tied to clients' mental and physical impairments. Both Rev. Scott and Ms. Worth can effectively articulate their needs to their formal caregivers. Their success depends on first being able to evaluate their needs and plan the tasks the aide must accomplish to meet those needs. Rev. Scott's plan for his homemaker aide includes a different kind of activity each week—shopping, washing, cleaning, and cooking. When his aide is competent, willing, and comes as scheduled (which is not always the case), his housekeeping needs are fulfilled.

In a similar manner, Ms. Worth knows what she needs, her medicine picked up at the pharmacy, for example, and plans accordingly. She calls her aide at home the night before to arrange her visit a little later in the morning, after the pharmacy opens. Her knowledge of the official role of aides—what tasks they are allowed to perform—influences which specific requests she makes. She knows that Anne is allowed to pick up her medicine, and this knowledge, together with Anne's willing attitude, leads her to make the appeal.

In Mrs. Starr's case, however, her encumbering attitudes are compounded by her mental and physical impairments. Because of her depression and anxiety, she is easily frustrated in her efforts to communicate. On days when her physical symptoms are more severe, she is even more averse to making these attempts:

I ain't much for telling folks what to do. It gets on my nerves real bad. . . . I don't know if she washed or not. I wasn't feeling too good. I didn't pay too much attention.

Because of her alcoholism and cognitive impairment, Mrs. Little is unable to evaluate her needs or to plan or organize her requests. In addition, she has difficulty sorting out who her aides are and when they come. Like Mrs. Starr, her incapacities merge with attitudes that deny the responsibility for, and doubt the efficacy of, such actions. She solicits only her most salient needs—her beer when the stash beside her bed is depleted or a meal from a fast-food restaurant. She never asks for help taking her medicine; nor does she plan ahead to have her clothes washed.

In some situations, when clients like Mrs. Little and Mrs. Starr are unable to organize and manage their services or communicate their needs, aides will assume a managerial role. Ms. Worth's aide, Anne, explains how she took charge of one client's care, developing a plan to meet the client's needs and even requesting extra time from her supervisor:

> Yes, I've got a patient I do that with. She's bedridden and used to live alone. Now her grandson is there. Now I would go in there and say, "What you want done?" and she would say, "Well, whatever you want. I don't have much money and I need some groceries." Well, to take clothes to the laundromat, have to do seven loads and takes full two hours to wash, dry, fold, and put away. So, it's like, "I can't go to the store the same day I do laundry. I can't cook you breakfast the same day I do laundry. This is what we're gonna do four times a week—Monday is an hour and a half day. I'll get you some breakfast. Then I'll go to the grocery store for you, little light things. Tuesday is two hours—laundry day. Make sure you keep out enough money from your check to do laundry, at least $10. That morning you get a bowl of cereal and a banana, and out the door I go. Then Wednesday, clean day—cook breakfast, wash dishes, clean the bathroom, mop." When you get somebody like that, and you go in and say, "What do you want done today," and they start naming off all this stuff they want you to do in an hour and a half, and they got four days with you—*that's* when you take control and say, "Now, we're gonna make out a schedule here." I had to ask for more time. This lady used to be three days a week. I went in and said, "Look, I can't go to the laundromat and those other things in an hour and a half." If you go over, you have to take it out of your next visit, which you shouldn't, as they [the clients] should get full time. That's when you go to your boss and you tell 'em that, and they're like, "O.K.," and in a couple of days, she's two hours. That extra thirty minutes, do I take back wet clothes or dry clothes?

Aides sometimes overstep the bounds clients define as appropriate initiative. As noted in Chapter 9, at times Ms. Worth is provoked when Anne performs tasks she, herself, has already done or believes are unnecessary. On several occasions, Mrs. Starr exploded when Lois overstepped her bounds.

## Client-Aide Bonds

In Chapter 10 we saw that some clients develop close personal relationships with their aides. In some cases the closeness of these bonds influences how client roles are enacted and the quality of care received.

Close relationships generate trust between clients and aides, often motivating clients to allow their aides to perform additional tasks like cashing checks and paying bills. Sometimes when close ties develop, clients are more effective at influencing their aides to provide the care they desire. The development of friendship between Rev. Scott and his homemaker aide, Mrs. Conner, enabled him to take more accurately her role in the caregiving process and encourage her to expand her services. Thomas, Franks, and Calonico also found accuracy in role-taking was increased when values were shared and high positive emotional bonds were present [14]. In Mrs. Starr's situation, however, being close to Vicky makes it harder for her to direct Vicky in the basic caregiving tasks. During many of Vicky's visits, Mrs. Starr focused more on the social aspects of the visit than on what caregiving tasks Vicky might accomplish.

## Other Strategies for Getting Help

Because these clients do not always ask for help and because requests do not always bring the desired results, some clients incorporate additional or alternative strategies into their client roles. As in their relationships with informal caregivers, these strategies often are designed to increase the benefits or reduce the costs to their aides.

## Giving Aides A Break

Some clients devise strategies they believe minimize for aides some of the more disagreeable aspects of their work. This objective gives Mrs. Starr an additional motive for performing herself the tasks she is able to do:

> I try to help her any way I can. I get the garbage up. I try not to leave any dishes in the sink for her. I wrap up my Dependens for

her. I got to use what sense I got and some of their's too. I try to make things easy for them 'cause I'm used to doin' for myself.

Ms. Worth regularly urges Anne to leave before the allotted time. By offering this reward to her aide, she hopes to benefit as well—by having an occasional extra service performed, one beyond the official job description of personal care aide, such as stopping by the store to buy milk:

> Monday she was so filled [had so many people to visit]. Those folks are crazy up there [at the office], all that extra work. I told her [Anne] I was going to run her out of here anyway. She got to help her ownself. Anne needs some rest too. I be looking out for Anne. If she finishes, I tell her to go on and sign the paper [time sheet] like she needs to. I done learnt I can ask you [to do special things]. You ain't got to tell 'em at the office. You help me, I'll help you.

Ms. Worth has discovered, however, that this strategy only works with a receptive partner. With another aide, it did not produce the desired effect:

> As many favors as I do for her, she doesn't want to go out of her way to try to help.

What is missing with this aide is Anne's willingness to expand her role to meet the unique needs of her client.

Ms. Worth is more successful than Mrs. Starr in getting her needs met. In part her success is related to her ability to take the role of her aide with greater accuracy. Following Goffman [15], role-taking can be used to control others' responses by pleasing them on their own terms. One's interpersonal skill or accuracy in role-taking determines the amount of influence one can exert. What she offers Anne (leaving early) is salient to Anne. Anne has numerous patients, about whose care she is very conscientious, and she also has a small child to pick up at day care at the end of her day. Mrs. Starr, on the other hand, performs for her aide those tasks that are reasonably easy and that are part of the normal homemaker aide's role. While she does not complain too loudly if Vicky takes a short nap, she gives her sporadic direction and regularly grumbles that her accomplishments are insignificant and the amount of time spent inadequate.

## Offering Money

Only Mrs. Starr regularly offers money to her paid helpers. She uses this strategy with her informal caregivers, and she believes that aides expect compensation as well. She ventures this payment, despite knowing such behavior is not officially sanctioned:

> I did something I shouldn't do. I was just showin' my appreciation. I know I ain't supposed to give it. They want you to put a piece of money in they hand. They lookin' for extra from these people that can't take care of themselves. They look for it. I know my race. If I feel like givin' 'em something, I do. They supposed to refuse it, but they don't have sense enough to. If you start givin' 'em something, they look for it. Everybody for self.

Although one time an aide rejected the money, "threw it back down on the table," another aide, and this same aide at a later date, verbalized at least tacit approval of monetary reward:

> They [other clients] don't offer you nothing. You'd think they'd offer a little something when you're trying to help.

Mrs. Starr established a pattern of paying Lois, her senior companion, for what she herself considered unpleasant chores or chores outside of Lois's job description. Her normal tendencies to offer money to Lois were buttressed by her view of the senior companion job, which paid less than minimum wage for part-time work, and her fear of losing Lois. While it was clear that Lois never requested payment, in Mrs. Starr's definition of the situation, the payment was necessary:

> Everybody lookin' for something. Claim they do it for charity. Guarantee they won't draw they hand back. I slip her something. It just tickles her to death. I give her some, what I felt like would make her happy. She would get me things, and I would pay her. I tried to give her a little along to keep her this way. She told me if they knew I was doing it, they would let her go. She knew I was giving her too much, but she didn't try to stop me. When I go to bank, I hand her a piece of money. I knowed it was too much. I had started giving her $40, $10 for little things she did. I just went crazy because I didn't want to lose her.

Because some aides accept payment and others expect it and because her values support it, Mrs. Starr routinely incorporates into her client role the strategy of offering money to her aides. For her, giving money is far better than "begging," that is, making requests. She is not going to do both:

> I won't beg folks and pay 'em, too.

## Praise, Cooperation, and Gratitude

Power in relationships can come from one's structural position in relation to another and from one's ability to control another based on interpersonal skill [14]. As in their interactions with informal caregivers, these participants possess different levels of interpersonal competence in their social exchanges with formal caregivers. Clients who have these skills are more successful in influencing their aides to perform the services they desire, even aides who are less willing. Rev. Scott has effective interpersonal skills and explains in the passage below his strategy for using them in interactions with Mrs. Conner, his homemaker aide:

> I find with some if you kind of brag on something they've done, it encourages them to want to do better, works better than talking in a derogatory way. Mrs. Conner had fixed some cornbread a time or two, and I kind of bragged on it, so when she went to grocery store, she got some flour, and one day she was back there cooking, and she made some biscuits, and those biscuits would crumble in your mouth, they were so tender, and so I bragged on her a little more about that, and so she made me some biscuits once in a while. Some clients are so unappreciative. Try to give them a hard time. I always try to say, "Thank you," when they get through. I think it works better than talking in a derogatory way about what somebody does. If you appreciate what they do, I think it works better. I guess I'm that way too. As I was saying, if you would have friends, you must be one.

In this encounter, Rev. Scott's strategy of positive reinforcement is designed to encourage Mrs. Conner's continued good service. Through past interactions with his aides, Rev. Scott has learned which strategies produce optimum results and which he should abandon:

> When Mrs. Conner started coming, I made the mistake of saying to her, Mrs. Pate [a former aide] did such and such, and she told me right quick, "I'm not Mrs. Pate," so I kind of eased off of that, and it turned out she was doing more things than Mrs. Pate.

Rev. Scott's influence is increased by his ability to take accurately the role of his aide and select the most effective strategy. By pleasing Mrs. Conner on her own terms, he gains greater power in the relationship and gets the services he desires. Thomas and his colleagues found in their study of role-taking between parents and children that persons occupying positions of less power tend to be more accurate role-takers than their more powerful counterparts [14]. We see parallels in relationships between clients and aides when clients use their positions of weakness to gain advantage.

Other research has confirmed the importance of client style in successful negotiation with aides [11]. Like Rev. Scott, Ms. Worth uses "Golden Rule" strategies to encourage and reward the kind of treatment she prefers. For her, this strategy means being nice, cooperative, and grateful:

> Don't expect that person to be the only somebody [her only regular helper] and you don't be nice to them. That client's gonna have to be nice to that aide. Just don't be uncooperative when people trying to do things for you. Some people, it looks like nothing you do is right, but still they can't help theyself. I know in my days and my times I have waited on people like that. It's the devil to wait on these folks, and they don't do nothing but try to be nasty. It's not right for the patient to always be doing them wrong. Some of 'em is so cruel and ungrateful that this aide can't do anything. I don't be contrary with my people. When you're so cruel, they make you suffer. We gonna get along. She don't dread coming, and I don't dread having her. That means more than money.

Ms. Worth has "waited on" people herself and adroitly takes her aide's role, using this information to mold her own behavior. She has a warm and friendly personality, often showing her affection for people with hugs and kind words, and she incorporates these traits into her client role. Many people, including her aides, like her and try to please her.

Mrs. Starr, on the other hand, is not socialized to give positive reinforcement and rarely praises her aides. Her choice of verbal abuse over the positive reinforcement Rev. Scott successfully employs brings her little satisfaction. The passage which follows, describing encounters with two different aides, illustrates her method of communicating—that being, as Rev. Scott would say, talking "in a derogatory manner:"

> Myrtice is runnin' me crazy. I'm gonna put a sign on my door, "Stay out." Me and Myrtice stays into it all the time. I said, "Myrtice, you don't never look under my bed to see if it's clean enough for me." [She would] turn on my television, open my refrigerator. "Don't open my refrigerator unless I tell you." I had to cuss her out all the time. This little young girl, I called her "dumb" the other day. I said, "I hate to tell you, but I can't hold it. It's coming out my mouth."

## Being Good

For certain clients the chosen strategy is simply to be compliant—to take what is offered and make few demands. This is the approach taken by Mrs. Washington:

> I try to be as good as I can. I try to get along with them as best I can because I'm handicapped.

Asymmetry in relationships with caregivers can be heightened when individuals are defined by themselves or others as sick and, thus, vulnerable and weak [8]. Mrs. Washington's passive behavior is influenced by feelings of powerlessness evoked by her dependency—behavior akin to that we identified in informal caregiving relationships.

## GOING TO THE SUPERVISOR

> *Don't lend 'em no money and don't have 'em searchin' in your belongings; don't feed 'em. If you ask 'em to do something and they say, "I don't do that," then report 'em.*
>
> Sally Finch

CCSP clients typically interact with workers in supervisory or managerial positions at times of regularly scheduled assessments and reviews and when they perceive and act to correct problems. These higher-level workers include case managers, RN's from the home health care agencies, assessors from the public health department, and representatives from other agencies that provide services. Clients are expected to convey their needs accurately and honestly to these workers and, to the extent they are able, to take actions to correct problems. All of these clients have needs that are not met, and/or they experience dissatisfaction with their services. Yet in many situations their complaints are not voiced, and no action is taken.

As in interactions with aides, how these clients enact their client roles with regard to formal workers in supervisory positions is determined by their attitudes and abilities and by their experiences—both of a lifetime and as care receivers. Their behavior toward supervisors is influenced by how they view their aides and the care they provide, how they interpret their rights and responsibilities as clients, and what their expectations are for the efficacy of their own actions. Taking corrective action requires knowledge of the formal program and its procedures and personnel and the skills to communicate needs effectively to workers in positions of authority. Seeking help from supervisors often means that clients have the "right" combination of abilities and supportive attitudes.

In some cases the effectiveness of clients' abilities are affected by various programmatic factors, such as workers who change frequently, the time of day a worker comes, or how long a particular problem continues. Many times it is how clients define the need for a particular service that is the critical element in whether action is taken.

## Knowing How

Going to the supervisor about a problem calls for specific knowledge and skills that not all clients possess. Some clients do not understand program information that has been conveyed to them or remember names of appropriate contact persons. Mrs. Little knows neither the names nor the phone numbers of her case manager, her RN, or even her aides who come every day. Although she keeps a list of "important" phone numbers close by, no formal workers are listed. She failed to notify the home health agency on her return home from one of her hospital stays because she did not know who to call or even *to* call. Consequently, she was without services for several days.

Client misunderstandings of programmatic organization also can interfere with attempts to redress problems. As noted, some clients are not completely aware of what services they are authorized to receive— what days aides come, what tasks they are expected to do, or the amount of time allocated for services. Difficulties arise simply in determining when a legitimate problem exists.

## Client Need

Clients who have alternative resources for care are less likely to complain when services are substandard or aides do not come. Mrs. Finch has never made complaining to the supervisor part of her client role. She might, however, *if* she had no other means of meeting her needs:

> I don't complain as long as I'm able. I might speak about it. If I ask and [they] don't do something—would have to be something I couldn't do.

Otherwise, she is willing to accept what might be a less-than-perfect service:

Rinse me off and go on about their business. Better than nothing
at all.

For similar reasons, Mr. Oliver does not call the supervisor when
his wife's aide fails to show up—because he is able to bathe her himself
or call the neighbor to fix her hair. When the problem is lack of
transportation to the ADR center, which provides the respite he so
badly needs, he notifies the agency without fail.

## Client-Aide Relationships

All of these clients demonstrate a certain loyalty toward, or sympathetic identification with, their aides, as if they are aligned with
them against the higher status workers in supervisory positions. They
understand the hardship of trying to survive with limited skills and a
low-paying job, and this understanding impedes their inclination to
take any action that might cause trouble for the worker. Mrs. Finch
expressed this viewpoint about an aide she believed had taken some
coasters from her apartment:

> I didn't want them to fire her. I felt sorry for her. She had two little
> children. I'm not going to make it hard on their jobs. It wasn't worth
> much no way. I don't want to hurt nobody. I've had hard times on
> the job. I don't call in no way (to the office) unless I call to see if
> somebody's coming. I felt sorry for her because she had children,
> but you can't go around people and take their stuff. No and that's a
> bad thing to do anyway.

Mrs. Little expressed similar feelings:

> I can't call 'em. Miss June [her RN] said to let her know. That's
> taking bread out of somebody's mouth. I'd hate for that to happen.

For Rev. Scott the attitude of the particular worker mitigates his
response:

> Well, I try not to report them unless I have to—if they make a
> move to try to get what they're supposed to do, done. If it was
> something that could be straightened out between me and that
> worker, I wouldn't want to report them as such because it could
> mean their job as such.

But when another aide seemed less willing to be helpful, he asked for a
replacement.

With the exception of Ms. Worth's aide, Anne, all of the aides also are African American. While a tacit loyalty to aides because of race is present in a number of these situations, only Mrs. Starr was explicit in her viewpoint:

> I don't want to break on my own color.

For Mrs. Starr, the more acceptable alternative to "reporting" an aide who does not show up on the appointed day is to call the aide at home and discuss the problem directly—a strategy not available to clients who do not have the knowledge or ability to make such contacts.

Feelings toward aides, however, can be complex, and while empathy is often present, in some situations clients fear retaliation by their aides, as stated by Mrs. Starr:

> If you squawk on 'em, they hate your guts. They know what they ain't doing. [If I] cause a whole lot of "rigamaro" and get 'em fired, they might come up and kill me.

Some fears are based on hearsay and some on reality. Mrs. Starr's apprehension is abetted by her encounter with an aide who was verbally and physically abusive:

> She had a habit of calling me crazy, [She would say] "She's going crazy, she's going crazy." She would raise her voice and bug her eyes. She hit me one time, and I hauled off and hit her right back. I'm actually scared of her.

Rev. Scott's retaliatory experience has made him more cautious:

> I let her have the money, thinking she'd do what she said. That time came, and she started giving me kind of a run around. I called the supervisor and asked for wage assignment on her. Well, they fired the lady, found out she was doing the same to others. Well, the other workers thought I was the cause of her getting fired and came in here with a nasty attitude doing things that were not becoming to what they should have been doing, talking nasty. One day I was notarizing something for someone, and she sat on the sofa instead of going in and washing dishes. When they left, she said, "You want me to wash your butt?"—like that, you know. I said, "We're just not going to have that kind of talk in here." As she rode off, I called the office and asked them not to send her back, but she came back that next day, and I wouldn't let her in here. That was after I talked to lady at the agency, and she said they would get me someone else, and that was the end of that. Sometimes they'll make it hard on

you. If you don't know who to talk to, you could get hurt. I didn't know about the rule about not lending them money; I don't usually lend money anyway. I just hated to see her go to jail when she's fixing to have the baby. She'd been coming here over two years, and I thought she was all right. I know people can, like, their attitude change, and they want to do mean things. I try to avoid such as that.

## Rights and Responsibilities

Rev. Scott had the skills to remedy his aide's retaliation—he knew whom to call and had the ability to communicate his needs. Rev. Scott also believes that it is his right to call the supervisor, and he expects the agency to be responsive. Some clients, however, have little faith that their appeals to higher authorities will produce the desired results. Ms. Worth expressed this viewpoint about trying to get her regular services started back after Medicare services terminated:

> I made up my mind I would do the best I could. I wouldn't say nothing. If you can't get nothing, be satisfied.

Mrs. Finch felt similarly powerless to request that her aide come early or to keep the same worker:

> I can't tell 'em when to send somebody because they do what they want to do. They won't do it for me. Look like they help everybody but poor me. I just take it like it is. Ain't nothing I can say. . . . Give those girls with cars those way out [out from the center of town]. Like the girl that was here before, she didn't have no car, but now she got a car, and they're likely to send her away. Then you got to start all over again. Just have to put up with it. They ain't gonna do nothing no way.

Mrs. Starr believes that voicing her complaints will not only fail to bring about the desired response, but may leave her in even worse shape:

> If I grumble too much, they won't let me have anybody at all. I asked her to send me somebody else. Ain't nothing I can do about it. They [RN supervisor and aide] in cahoots together.

On the other hand, a successful experience can encourage a typically reluctant client to seek future remedies. Once when Rev. Scott failed to complain about an unsatisfactory worker, the supervisor sensed a problem, encouraged him to discuss it with her, and made a satisfactory response. Because of her action, he has been more willing to assert himself. Even when assertive, however, clients' actions are not always effective. Rev. Scott notes one disappointing attempt:

> I reported [the aide's suspicious behavior] and that I couldn't prove it, but I wasn't too much for her being my aide, and that's when I say it seemed that, that was as good as they wanted, and they said, "Oh, she's the right person for him," and let her stay here two years. Just had to deal with it the best I could. If the supervisor don't believe what somebody else say, want to take side with the worker, then that makes it bad.

Client doubts about the efficacy of their actions to correct problems are likely rooted also in their own life experiences being poor, African American, and, more recently, disabled. Mrs. Washington explains her failure to assert herself in terms of her dependency:

> I didn't tell 'em. I just let 'em go on. I'm dependent. I can't be too choicy.

When persons of authority within the formal system are also white, feelings of powerlessness can be heightened. Although two out of the three case managers participating in this study are black, all of the RN supervisors and assessors are white. The RN supervisors are the persons of authority who have the most direct contact with clients concerning their aide services, and it is clear that clients are ever-mindful of status differences.

Being of the same race does not guarantee that clients will feel more powerful in relationships with higher status persons. An opinion often voiced was that black persons who have attained positions of authority often "act worse than white people," a perspective shared by Mrs. Starr:

> Colored and white all is messy. Some of the whites is just as mean as the colored. Why do our race of people do such things. Poor folks catch the devil.

For her, being poor is a greater burden in such encounters than being African American.

Clients' beliefs about their abilities to act effectively in interactions with supervisors are influenced also by their understanding of the formal care system. Mrs. Starr's attitude that she has little power relative to her case manager is based both on her past frustrating experiences trying to get help from her and on her own failure to understand the program and the case manager's formal role:

> Why didn't you tell me all that? I ain't for playing with. I didn't know what she was. I didn't have a caseworker. She said she was my caseworker. Why didn't she tell me? I told her I had a white caseworker that was nice. They ain't gonna do a damn thing anyway. I didn't want to hurt her feelings 'cause I'd have to go to her again. She never come out here. She never call me. I just quit bothering with Janet. I don't call her much. When I call on Wednesday, she's so busy she can hardly talk to you. If I call, "Gone for the day." I just want you [the researcher] to call and see what kind of tale she tell you. She don't think I'm sick. She don't come out here but once a year [in reality she came out every 3 months], putting on all those two cents airs. I've been knowin' her quite a while. It's just a lot of apple salt. I knew she ain't got time to fool with me. She's so anxious to put me in a nursing home. She can call me every now and then.

Rev. Scott's much more accurate understanding of the program affords him more realistic expectations that allow him to be assertive when appropriate:

> Of course if I get the feeling they [the home health agency] trying to get around doing the services or make promises and don't do 'em, then I know that I can call Mrs. LaRossa [the case manager]. I would think I should first call the supervisor and see what they would do about it, and if I don't get any answers there, then I would do otherwise. Well, I really haven't had any problems to be calling her. I called her about some other matters when I was trying to get some help with some music last summer, but [if] something go wrong, I think I feel free to let her know.

Rev. Scott's actions are reinforced by the responsiveness of his case manager, who has taken a special interest in him, even bringing the pianist from her church out to play for him.

## Problems in the System

A variety of programmatic complexities or constraints impede clients' abilities to identify problems accurately and take corrective action. Lack of continuity in workers affects clients' knowledge of who is who, who is supposed to do what, and when services are scheduled. Mrs. Washington explains how frequent changes in aides confuse her:

> They don't ever send one back. Different one coming every time. Was coming once a month, but now she says every two weeks. I won't know till they come back. I get confused too. I forgets a whole lot too.

Mrs. Washington had five different regularly scheduled aides during the twelve-month study period, in addition to those who filled in during absences. Mrs. Finch weathered similar capricious service:

> You know what I'm going to do? Write it down. It gets me so confused. Now Barbara come here, and I got her name. Then she might go, and here come another one. They stay two or three weeks, and here come another. They get you confused.

Mrs. Finch is referring to her personal care aides, whose names she has difficulty remembering, but she is able to name neither her case manager nor the RN supervisor from the home health agency. While no case managers assigned to these clients changed during the course of this study, typically their contacts with clients are limited—generally adhering to the required three-month reviews—the experience of four of these seven clients. The other three clients had only one additional contact during the research period. Clients have difficulty becoming acquainted with RN supervisors, who change even more frequently than aides and, when no skilled services are required, visit only every two months.

The strategy of writing down the various workers' names was used by several clients and is a plausible one for Mrs. Finch—she has the necessary skills, and she has a special chest in her living room where she keeps important papers. For a client like Mrs. Washington, this strategy is less likely due to her poor eyesight and to the general chaos of her living situation—visitors coming in and out and the disarray of her belongings. In her case, she keeps her critical papers in her pocketbook, the very one that disappeared with her nighttime burglar.

Sometimes it is a program malfunction that prevents clients' actions to correct problems. Rev. Scott often failed to notify the agency about one aide's regular absences because he never knew until too late whether or not she would actually arrive. He explains:

> Well, the lady was coming so late in the day that I didn't know she was not coming until so late the office would be closed at that time. Like on Friday, she hadn't come, June 28th. That Thursday before the 4th was the last day she came. Nobody came on Friday. I didn't

know till too late to call. The next Tuesday leading up to the 4th [on Wednesday], I kept thinking somebody was coming. So Thursday morning I called, and they sent somebody out, but they didn't come back Friday.

* * * * *

Our data show that the client role is composed of six specific elements— 1) assessing needs for care, 2) setting goals for care, 3) developing a care plan, 4) communicating needs for care, 5) evaluating care, and 6) taking actions to correct problems. While a number of these elements correspond to services provided by the Community Care Services Program, clients often take on these tasks themselves in the ongoing process of care.

A number of reasons account for clients' continuing involvement in assessing their own needs. Fluctuations in chronic conditions lead to changes in needs clients may have communicated at one time to an assessor, case manager, or supervisor. Clients also sometimes fail to communicate their needs accurately to those in supervisory positions. They may not know what type of help is available, not know what they need, know that what they *really* need (that is, an unavailable service or a body that works better) is not possible, or may doubt a satisfactory response to their actions.

Clients attempt to participate in planning their own care for some of the same reasons that they assess their own needs. That is, if the professionals cannot properly evaluate their needs, it is likely that the resulting care plan will be inadequate. Whether or not clients are able to develop their own care plan is dependent on their knowledge of the program and their intellectual skills.

Although each client's plan of care is routinely communicated to aides by the RN supervisor, as a rule it is based on regularly scheduled annual assessments by public health personnel and on three-month reviews by case managers. Unless clients initiate other contacts, no other assessments are performed, except when skilled RN services are provided. In situations where RN's regularly visit, an official care plan is sometimes changed in response to client needs, but official plans can be problematic.

While asking for needed help is sometimes necessary to get the care desired, we found in certain situations clients are unwilling or unable to communicate their needs for care to their aides. In some cases clients develop additional strategies designed to persuade their aides to provide needed care or to make providing care more rewarding. The success of such strategies depends in part on clients having the resources necessary to influence their aides, but success depends also on the willingness of aides to be influenced.

In many instances clients do not incorporate the final element—taking actions to correct problem situations—into their client roles. These actions can involve both aides and supervisors, and with both levels of workers, clients often feel powerless to correct problems. Sometimes this perception is accurate.

None of these clients is able to make each element of the ideal client role a part of his or her unique, personalized version of the role. For each element, specific resources and attitudes are necessary prerequisites for role performance, many of which are lacking among this group of clients. But it is clear that the presence or absence of these elements is a significant factor in the relative satisfaction of clients with their formal care. Thornton and Nardi suggest that effective role performance comes only after individuals have modified their roles to fit themselves—have taken their own unique abilities, skills, personalities, values, and beliefs and made them a part of role performance [6]. In the view of these authors, optimum satisfaction is derived when performers are able to fuse themselves with their roles. Only then is meaning given to role performance. We would argue that the more elements clients are able to incorporate into their roles as clients and the more fully they adapt to or embrace the client role, the greater will be their success in having their goals met.

Corbin and Strauss discussed the fragile and complex equilibrium of the long-term care situation and the need for "making arrangements"—a process that caregivers use to reach and maintain agreements for carrying out caregiving tasks [16]. Arrangements are arrived at through negotiations between the care receiver and the various caregivers. Because of the tenuous nature of many home care situations, these authors compared managing care in the home to an acrobatic act. Arrangements must be both standing and temporary and must be renegotiated on a regular basis. It is these kinds of arrangements that often fall through unless the client or, in the Olivers' case, the informal caregiver, is able to take a major role. Corbin and Strauss emphasized the value of structural resources and supportive agents for managing care in the home. We found that in many situations the personal attributes of the care receivers are more critical than those of their informal caregivers.

In the final chapter we consider the implications of our findings for the development of long-term care policies that will help clients attain their goals. We offer strategies for providing care that enable providers to gain greater understanding of the care receiver's situation, to take into account the care receiver's point of view, and to build their programs around the goals and the roles that clients prefer.

## REFERENCES

1. P. Dressel, *The Service Trap*, Charles C. Thomas, Springfield, Illinois, 1984.
2. C. Maslach, The Client Role in Staff Burnout, *Journal of Social Issues, 34*, pp. 111-124, 1978.
3. R. H. Turner, Unanswered Questions in the Convergence between Structuralist and Interactionist, in *Micro-Theory*, H. J. Helle and S. N. Eisenstadt (eds.), Vol. 2, Sage Publications, Inc., London, 1985.
4. S. Stryker and R. Serpe, Commitment, Identity Salience, and Role Behavior: Theory and Research Example, in *Personality, Roles, and Social Behavior*, W. Ickes and E. S. Knowles (eds)., Springer-Verlag, New York, pp. 199-218, 1982.
5. R. Turner, Role Taking: Process Versus Conformity, in *Human Behavior and Social Process*, A. Rose (ed.), Houghton Mifflin, Boston, 1962.
6. R. Thornton and P. Nardi, The Dynamics of Role Acquisition, *American Journal of Sociology, 80*, pp. 870-883, 1975.
7. J. A. Altholz and M. L. Duggar, *Mobilizing Community Resources: A Case Management Perspective*, Georgia Department of Human Resources, Office of Aging, 1985.
8. S. W. Bloom and R. Wilson, Patient-Practitioner Relationships, in *Handbook of Medical Sociology*, H. E. Freeman, S. Levine, and L. G. Reeder (eds.), Prentice-Hall, Englewood Cliffs, New Jersey, pp. 275-296, 1972.
9. P. Feldman, Work Life Improvements for Home Care Workers: Impact and Feasibility, *The Gerontologist, 33*:1, pp. 47-54, 1993.
10. M. MacAdam, Home Care Reimbursement and Effects on Personnel, *The Gerontologist, 33*:1, pp. 55-63, 1993.
11. N. N. Eustis, R. A. Kane, and L. R. Fischer, Home Care Quality and the Home Care Worker: Beyond Quality Assurance as Usual, *The Gerontologist, 33*:1, pp. 64-73, 1993.
12. R. Surpin and F. Grumm, Building the Home Care Triangle: Clients and Families, Paraprofessionals and Agencies, *Caring*, pp. 6-15, 1990.
13. E. P. Stoller and S. J. Cutler, Predictors of Use of Paid Help Among Older People Living in the Community, *The Gerontologist, 33*:1, pp. 31-40, 1993.
14. D. Thomas, D. Franks, and J. Calonico, Role-taking and Power in Social Psychology, *American Sociological Review, 37*, pp. 128-137, 1972.
15. E. Goffman, *The Presentation of Self in Everyday Life*, Anchor Books, New York, 1959.
16. J. M. Corbin and A. Strauss, Making Arrangements: The Key to Home Care, in *The Home Care Experience*, J. F. Gubrium and A. Sankar (eds.), Sage Publications, Inc., Newbury Park, California, pp. 59-74, 1990.

# Part IV
# Conclusion

# CHAPTER
12

# What Does It Mean?

*I don't grieve—I just try.*
Irene Worth

Sometimes nothing helps. It is well to remember that fact when dealing with people who are very old and very frail. Often the many complex problems besetting our seven informants appeared overwhelming. Sometimes they were. By most measures, Mrs. Little is a pitiful person in horrendous circumstances. She has outlived her body and lost contact with her family. All that remains, unfortunately for her, is her mind, although most of the time she seems determined to deaden with alcohol all consciousness of the misery in which she finds herself. Yet, she persists. Even through her alcoholic haze, she controlls her bed, and in so doing, her tiny sphere. Malnutrition has weakened her grasp on life and shortened her reach, but, determined that her reach will exceed her grasp, she extends herself and her span of control by fashioning a clothes hanger into her "wire" with which she pushes and pulls her necessities into their proper orbits. Amidst the horror of sickness, isolation, alcoholism, incontinence, malnutrition, poverty, and being cared for by strangers, she refuses to give up.

At the other end of this narrow spectrum is Irene Worth. She is spry in mind and spirit, if not in body. A lifetime of physical deformity and disability may have taught her the lessons she would need as her age further impaired her abilities. Whether by better fortune or better choices, Ms. Worth has found avenues of compensation to fill the gaps in her old age resources. When she said, "I don't grieve—I just try," she explained her most successful strategy for surviving dependence. Her ability to adapt to her circumstances, to make the best of a bad situation, usually allows Ms. Worth to have her needs met in ways that preserve her independence. She is, of course, not independent, but her

235

dependence is weighed against that of others less able and redefined as independence of a sort—one no less precious merely because it is not complete. This pragmatic attitude, supported by other psychological, social, spirtitual, intellectual, and material resources, is essential for her success. Each of the other six older persons share Ms. Worth's value and goal of independence, and each—even Mrs. Little—is able, through their own resources and techniques, to manufacture a personal version of autonomy. If there is a pervasive mindset among our seven informants, retaining some degree of autonomy is it.

It is against this stunningly simple, yet irresistible reality that we attempt to outline the lessons of our observations—first for home care practice and then for research.

## IMPLICATIONS FOR HOME CARE PRACTICE

In her review of home care research, Chappell suggested that studies of the experience of home care, such as ours, are more relevant to practice issues than to broad matters of policy [1]. Just so. Our analysis certainly yields more insights for program planners than for policymakers, though some ideas are important enough that they may warrant consideration of a policy shift. On the other hand, our findings do not always imply a specific, achievable program change. We sometimes describe problems without being able to identify solutions. We do make suggestions for small and large changes we feel would enhance the quality of care. Many of these ideas are not new—some are even cliches—but all are supported by our data, many for the first time in a minority population. Taken on a large scale, the impact of even the smallest change could be great.

We undertook this study to learn something about how elderly African Americans live through disability and dependency. We wanted to know how their experiences might parallel or diverge from those of older whites. Many of our findings lead us to believe, at least for this special population, that cultural differences are slight and the degree of overlap quite substantial. In the discussion that follows we give special attention to the few instances we noted where race seems to make a difference. Otherwise, based on our examination of the literature we believe the experience of home care is largely race-neutral and that many of our observations about these African Americans could apply as well to elderly, disabled whites.

It has become common to evaluate any health care system according to the three basic principles of access, cost, and quality. Other studies have focused either on access to home care or its cost relative to institutional care. Quite a few have tried to gauge the impact of care on some desired outcome for the recipient, a way of judging the effectiveness, and possibly the quality, of the care provided. While we did not undertake this study to evaluate any of these dimensions of home care, our findings bear most directly on the issue of quality. In the following pages, based on those findings, we make specific recommendations for improving the quality of care. These recommendations pertain to the clients, their caregivers—both informal and formal—and the system of care.

## Recommendations about the Clients

1. *Home care should be provided in a way that recognizes and takes into account the client's definition of high quality care.*

Our findings suggest that, for these individuals, high quality care possesses three features: 1) empowerment of the client; 2) an individualized approach; and 3) a caring attitude. By empowerment, we mean actions that permit clients to perceive themselves as effectual and maintain a sense of control, independence, and autonomy. Often the participants complained about aides, family members, friends, or other helpers who tried to "boss" them, who thought they knew better what the care receivers needed than the care receivers did themselves. While we recognize that none of us always knows fully our own needs, and we appreciate the inherent difficulty of delivering care and autonomy at the same time, we firmly believe and we recommend that:

2. *The guiding tenet of all home care should be the preservation and enhancement of the client's independence, to the maximum degree possible.*

Athough this concept may appear obvious, it has not always been adhered to, at least not in ways our findings would support. Several other investigators have reported that the desire for more control and choice in their care arrangements is a strong theme among older persons receiving long-term care [2-6]. As noted throughout the earlier chapters, independence is the overriding value of the individuals portrayed here, and it is largely their own personal resources—however depleted—that allow them to maintain the independence they still possess, both in taking care of their own needs and in maintaining supportive relationships. It seems just as obvious that independence would be enhanced by increasing those personal resources.

This could be done in several ways. As Weber observed long ago, one's personal resources inhere in the possession of power, prestige, or property [7]. Power in this context involves the ability to decide one's fate, to make choices. The association between the availability of choice and client satisfaction with care among the participants in our study was universally strong. Given the impaired state of these clients, however, it may be unrealistic to expect them to be able to know everything they need to know and to make every decision. As Hennessy argued, the goal should be a sharing of power between care receivers and caregivers [6]. We have observed that these seven informants often functioned as informal managers of their own care, since the case management function often seemed to operate at a distance. This would seem the ideal arena for such shared power and responsibility, provided the professional case manager were aware of the client's desire and ability to share this role and were trained to accommodate it. Thus, we recommend that:

3. *Home health care should be provided in a way that supports and utilizes the client's role as informal care manager.*

Choice without knowledge, however, is an empty promise. Clients must be provided with an array of information in order to exercise power effectively. They must be apprised of their rights under the program of care to be provided. They need to know how the system works, whom their aides are and what they are supposed to do (and not do), whom to call if they have a problem, and that they have a right to "have it their way." We found that no client knew all this information, and some of them were completely unaware of any of it. Sabatino pointed out that providers and clients have different value orientations about the rights of clients [3]. Clients are more interested in general civil rights and do not like the adversarial connotation of "rights" within the context of care, preferring to focus instead on their "expectations" of caregivers. The home care industry, as a whole, does a poor job of conveying this information in a way that insures the client understands and can use it later. Sabatino suggested that such expectations could be reconceptualized as the client's "management skills" and that they might be taught through peer support groups. While the notion of support groups for home care clients is certainly a novel one, we believe they could function as a means of socialization to the new role of home care client. They might also be an effective mechanism for teaching or enhancing the skills the client needs to enact the role of informal care manager: communication and negotiation. Certainly, not every client could function appropriately in such a role, but most could improve on the job they already are performing with mixed results, and nearly all could benefit from the attempt.

Since the goal is to enlarge and enhance the client's role, they also should be told their responsibilities as care receivers—to give clear guidance to caregivers about their preferences, to monitor services provided, to report service lapses and problems, and to understand and appreciate the limitations and difficulties imposed on the caregivers by the system. We recognize the forces that could constrain such an ambitious effort, including the ever-increasing pool of unserved clients, the continuing shortage of resources, the ideology of paternalism that dominates the health and social services professions, and the inherent role conflict such an approach could present to practitioners trained in those fields. We wonder, but cannot say, whether the race of these clients may make them particularly vulnerable to paternalism and the assumption of managerial incompetence by their formal caregivers. We reiterate, nevertheless, our strong conclusions, based on the data presented, that many clients would be responsive to such a strategy and competent to learn it and that both their perceived and actual quality of care would be improved as a result.

Another means of empowering these clients would be to increase their material resources. A popular contemporary definition of the "Golden Rule" holds that whoever has the gold makes the rules. Under current policies, the delivery system limits choices; clients have no gold and, thus, no power. These are poor people who can barely provide for their basic shelter, food, and clothing needs. Few have even a few extra dollars for elective spending on items or services that might increase their well-being and their independence. We recommend, therefore, that:

4. *Direct financial support for the elderly poor should be increased.*

Additional money would enable clients to secure additional help, as Rev. Scott does in paying Deacon Pate $40 a month to provide personalized transportation and assistance with other routine business. He is thus able to avoid the agency-provided transportation service he finds so tiring. If Mrs. Finch could afford it, she might hire someone to provide the help she needs getting around the large county hospital when she goes for her regular appointments. As it is, her disposable income is spent paying her sister-in-law to do her shopping and banking. Additional cash also could be used to purchase or repair appliances, to buy more prepared foods, which would decrease the need for food preparation and increase nutritional status, or to purchase non-medical assistive devices not covered by Medicare or Medicaid. Although a variety of medically-related home care devices to compensate for various handicaps are now readily available and free of charge from Medicare and Medicaid—e.g., portable toilets, walkers, and manual wheelchairs—some devices require a copayment to purchase. The electrically-powered three-wheeled scooter that Mrs. Little acquired—

at a time past the point she was able to use it because of the bureaucratic process involved—required a $30 per month co-payment to cover her total cost share of $600. Additional problems arise because some individuals are not aware of what devices are available, and some are not educated in their use. Once Mrs. Little did acquire her cart, she received one introductory instructional session and then was on her own, an uneasy situation for her. Thus, an educational component to accompany this type of assistance—possibly an annual, or as-needed, visit from an occupational therapist—could facilitate the use of devices. The therapist would have to be patient with attitudes resistant to changing a lifetime of self-care and housekeeping patterns.

Other, less direct methods of increasing the resources of these dependent persons also could be beneficial. A priority should be home maintenance and improvement. Programs are needed to bring homes up to minimal standards of safety and sanitation. For seven years, rain has leaked into Mrs. Little's bedroom because she cannot afford more than occasional patchwork repairs. Although she applied for assistance from a program that does such repairs, she has been on the waiting list for over a year. Another prime need of our participants is for improvement of the handicapped accessibility of their homes. Such alterations would enhance, and in some cases allow for the first time, ease of mobility around the interior of residences and to the world beyond. With this type of amendment, Mrs. Oliver and Mrs. Washington could use their bathrooms independently in their wheelchairs, and Rev. Scott could ride down to the street in his power chair. Someone could push Mrs. Little around her neighborhood or to the store to pick out her own groceries, and she even might be able to continue attending the ADR program that she loves so much.

In addition to improving mobility, a myriad of other changes—such as adjusting the heights of counters and bathroom fixtures and installing different kinds of door handles—could be made to facilitate caring for basic needs. Washing machines and dryers in the homes of Rev. Scott and Mrs. Little would increase the efficiency of aides. Mrs. Little's aide does no laundry, a service she badly needs, and Rev. Scott's sometimes consumes her entire time going to the laundromat. In many cases, the cost of such improvements would be minimal compared to the benefits received in augmented independence. The accessibility of highrise apartments could be improved with relative ease as well. A simple change like automatic electric doors would encourage Mrs. Finch to go to the vegetable truck herself, and an adjustment in the door sill would permit Mrs. Starr to propel herself out the door with ease to empty her own trash. As it is, Mrs. Starr is fearful that the effort of getting over the high sill will make her fall. A wheelchair-accessible kitchen would decrease considerably the stress of cooking for her, a task she is determined to continue performing independently.

While indirect support often is helpful, direct financial support is preferred because of the greater degree of control it grants over how needed care is provided. Money confers both status and choice. For people who have functional disabilities, increased income is preferable to programs offering alternative benefits that require additional effort by the recipient. The food stamp program, for example, furnishes coupons that must be redeemed for the actual food vouchers. This extra step in the process of procuring groceries necessitates additional assistance from others or, at the very least, money for taxi fare. It represents, as well, an entirely different bureaucratic system, with all the attendant frustrations and barriers. For these reasons, only two of these seven individuals participated in the food stamp program, although all of them were financially eligible and often needed additional money for food. For them, the costs of participation outweighed the possible benefits.

It may seem willfully naive, but we believe the most certain way to increase the autonomy of these clients is to increase their SSI benefits. While it is true that SSI is indexed to inflation (as is Social Security) and so cannot fall behind the cost of living, neither can it push ahead. Incomes for recipients may no longer be fixed, but their relative economic position is. If a person is poor, she or he will stay that way. There is, of course, no question that SSI is a necessary and welcome source of economic support for millions who, without it, would be far worse off. It simply does not provide the level of support necessary for these impaired individuals to meet their own needs and live a decent life.

After empowerment, a second important way of supporting the client would be to make a greater effort to provide individualized care. Although these clients share certain basic problems, their needs vary both in kind and in priority, as do their alternatives for informal support. In addition, we found enormous variation in situations over time, with gradual declines mixed in with collapses, rallies, and successful rehabilitation. All too often, our participants were compelled to fit a Procrustean Bed presented either by the program or inflexible aides. As Cantor and Chichin have argued, care plans must be flexible to accommodate both sudden and gradual changes [8]. Aides should be more versatile, with the clients controlling, to the highest degree possible, their own services. In those situations where informal care is minimal and clients' needs great, as with Mrs. Little, the limited role and time allowed the home health aide is of questionable value, particularly when the client has attitudes strongly resistant to traditional health care. We recommend, therefore:

5. *Home care clients should receive services as closely tailored as possible to their individual needs and tastes.*

In addition to the principal goal of independence, we found that the outcomes clients seek from their home care experiences cover three general areas of need—basic physical care, emotional care, and social integration. Data show that aides' effectiveness in achieving these outcomes depends, in the client's view, on whether they perform their tasks according to the client's wishes. Clients want their needs met, but they define the *way* a task is done as part of those needs. Client satisfaction seems to depend as much on the quality of care as on the quantity—or even the fact—of the care.

It is also clear that the roles clients are allowed to take in the formal caregiving process also can have a major impact on their satisfaction with that process. How these client roles are defined and played depends largely on the resources clients have for performing the role, on the attitudes they have toward the care they receive, and the expectations they have for the results of their actions. As in relationships with informal caregivers, clients develop strategies to maximize their benefits and minimize their costs, and, to the best of their abilities, they create the role that serves their caregiving interests. We found that the ideal client role is composed of five elements or tasks: 1) assess need, 2) develop plan of care, 3) communicate plan to aide, 4) persuade aide to carry out plan, and 5) take action to correct problems. When successfully performed, this role resembles the role of case manager. The client role, therefore, is actively "made," not passively played, as often assumed. Under the best circumstances, clients can find meaning and satisfaction in the interactons required to participate in decisions about their own care. As noted previously in Recommendation 2, we strongly urge program planners and managers to consider ways of allowing clients to assume a greater degree of responsibility for planning and directing their own care. Such a strategy would require a highly individualized approach but would yield greater benefits in terms of the client's evaluation of the quality of care.

The third criterion of quality care, as seen by clients, is that the caregiver display a caring attitude. This finding echoes those of Eustis and her colleagues [2, 9]. Aides can be placed into three categories based on how they carry out the process of care—those that have an expanded role, going beyond what is required, those who perform only the expected tasks, and those who perform less than is required by agency guidelines. Clients explain these variations in an aide's performance as dependent on whether or not aides care about their clients and about their jobs. By the clients' definition, an aide who does more than is required or tries to do her tasks according to the client's preferences, is caring; one who does less or does things contrary to the client's wishes, is not. This utterly logical, yet crucial, step seems to us the simplest—if not the easiest—to enact of all our recommendations.

6. *Aides should perform tasks as and when the client prefers, to the extent possible.*

## Recommendations about the Caregivers

### Informal Caregivers

Our informants vary in the relative significance of their informal support. In the two cases where spouses act as primary caregivers, this support is sufficient to care for most basic needs; in the other cases, informal support is still critical, but much less extensive. In each case, needs for additional care remain, and it is to fill these gaps that formal care is provided. Much has been written in the last few years about the need to support informal caregivers. "Who is caring for the caregivers?" is a question often heard. Our data confirm this as an important issue, but offer few positive solutions. We can say from our observations that the goal of partnership between informal and formal care providers is not a reality among these clients. Except for Mr. Oliver, little contact of any sort was seen or reported between agencies or aides and family members or neighbors. To begin to make this phantom partnership materialize, we would suggest:

7. *The principle of individualized care should take account of informal support resources and needs as well as those of the client.*

In addition, regular consultation between formal and informal caregivers could only enhance understanding and inform wise decisions by all involved. In the final analysis, however, perhaps the best hope for supporting informal caregivers is to provide more and better support and care to the client.

### Formal Caregivers

Much also has been written about the difficulties associated with the home care worker's job [2, 10, 11]. It is physically and emotionally demanding and requires technical skill, good judgment, an ethical sense, and a caring attitude. And the pay is lousy. Small wonder that absenteeism, customer complaints, and turnover are high. Everyone

244 / SURVIVING DEPENDENCE

agrees that aides are overworked, undertrained, and underpaid. While our focus was on the clients and not the workers, we believe that any improvement for the aide will be an improvement for the client. Therefore, we recommend:

8. *The position of home care worker should be enhanced through better training, higher status, higher pay, and a reduced client load.*

Recognizing the tinge of fantasy associated with this recommendation, we wish to stress its clear potential for high-yield dividends in both quality of care and cost saving. A better trained worker is more professional, more efficient, and more effective. Increased professionalism, if supported by higher salaries (i.e., higher than slightly above the minimum wage), likely would lead to a lower turnover rate and higher occupational status. Pride in one's work and job satisfaction are literally a recipe for quality. If clients perceived that their caregivers were professionals receiving adequate compensation for their work, it might increase their willingness to make demands [2].

Lest the point be lost, we should remember the ironic similarities between the home care workers we observed and their clients. By continuing to employ mainly semi-skilled workers, by paying them little and providing few health or pension benefits, and by affording them little meaning and satisfaction in their work, we are quite literally creating the poor, disabled, older home care clients of the future. Our welfare system is feeding on itself. It is insuring that this chain-letter of dependency will be forwarded to the next generation. The expense of improvement is dwarfed by that of doing nothing.

Another program change that could improve the working conditions of the aides—and probably clients' services—would be to reduce the client load. Because the job is so physically and emotionally draining, it is unrealistic to think that even the best of aides can minister to as many different clients as they do on a daily basis and still provide competent care, with a willing attitude, to each one. They need *time* to care.

Finally, we invoke Hennessy's notion of "shared power" as a strategy for empowering workers and clients alike [6]. As we argue above in the interest of client control and independence, so must aides gain a feeling of autonomy if they are to become—or approach—professional status. How this could be done requires more than facile generalizations. It seems clear that input to care plans and plan modifications must not be limited to case managers or RNs or even clients. Front-line workers, properly trained and motivated, could and should provide valuable information in these efforts. It seems equally clear that empowering the disenfranchised would not diminish those with power but in fact could make the whole system more effective.

## Recommendations about the Program

In addition to increasing the resources of clients and caregivers, other reccommendations can be directed at improving care programs. Our first observation about the Community Care Services Program is painfully obvious to all who labor within it and to every student who has struggled to understand it: it is mind-numbingly complex. Different functions not only are assigned to different individuals, but to different agencies. One agency determines financial eligibility. Another agency determines functional eligibility and devises a care plan. A third selects and oversees a fourth agency to implement it. Additional (non-CCSP) services may be provided by a fifth, sixth, or even a seventh, organization or funding source. Sometimes services are provided by CCSP agencies but paid for by Medicare. An entirely different agency—the Georgia Division of Aging Services—is charged with policy development and general oversight of the program. This is a blueprint for confusion. Responsibility is too diffused among the players. Too many different types of aides are being paid by too many different organizations to perform too many similar tasks, and they are being directed and supervised by too many different individuals. Such a system inevitably creates service gaps and overlaps. The unconvinced should return to the opening pages of Chapter 8—and take a compass.

One is reminded of the old saying about the camel being actually a horse designed by a committee. CCSP came into being at the hands of a task force of professionals and community leaders representing, among others, the range of interests that eventually would stake out a piece of the action: the Division of Aging Services, the Department of Medical Assistance (Medicaid), the Division of Public Health, the Department of Family and Children's Services, area agencies on aging, local aging network providers, and private home care providers. Although this is a classic approach to planning a new program—especially one likely to infringe on established turf—it largely determined the ultimate camel-shaped structure of the program. To its credit, program overseers have recognized at least some of the ill effects of the program's complexity and recently moved to combine two of the aide categories—the personal care and homemaker aides—into one, a "personal support aide." The program model, unfortunately remains as complicated—and as pernicious for clients—as when it was created. We recommend:

9. *The structure of the Community Care Services Program should be simplified and made more client-centered.*

Case management has emerged as the intervention mode of choice in the provision of extended, continuing care to chronically impaired clients in community settings. To be effective, this method must be able to meet the unique needs of clients at any point as well as to ensure continuity of services over time, a highly complex function requiring a variety of roles and skills. While highly valued as an intervention method for providing long-term care services, case management lacks definitional consensus and conceptual clarity [12]

In Georgia's Community Care Services Program, case management is considered a management and administrative service that involves planning, linking, coordinating, and evaluating the delivery of direct services to clients [13]. The case manager is expected to know and understand the client's situation and preferences and to personalize the system. Case managers have the responsibility to respond to the "whole person"—to take into account the medical, psychological, social, economic, and environmental needs of the client. Services should be appropriate to clients' changing situations, and a major goal of case management is the maximization of client independence. Case managers are cautioned against believing they know the best interests of the client better than the client does. They are encouraged to build relationships with clients based on understanding, trust, and respect and to make every attempt to involve clients in the decision-making process, thereby giving them a sense of control.

While the goals of CCSP are laudable and embody many of the same goals we found our participants to value, in many instances the role of the case manager did not live up to these expectations. Rothman suggested that without adequate funding and supportive services, case management can be used to project only the illusion of responsible caregiving [12]. We believe this often to be the case in Georgia. With case loads ranging from 70-100 persons, how can case managers be expected to know and understand their clients and their situations or to develop relationships of trust and respect. With the exception of Rev. Scott, clients were visited by their case managers only at the mandated three-month intervals. Ruby Washington's case manager was never aware that Mr. Jones was her husband, believing him to be only a neighborhood helper. Mrs. Little's case manager was unaware of any of Mrs. Little's health crises and hospitalizations. In a few instances additional telephone contacts were made, but at the client's initiation. We therefore make the following recommendations:

10. *Case managers' case loads should be reduced to a level that allows more frequent contact with clients and thus greater knowledge and understanding of clients.*

If caseloads were reduced, the case manager would be in a better position to provide on-going evaluation and review of the client's needs and might have the time to begin the long process of bridging the cultural gulf that lies between them and their clients. Further:

11. *The assessment component of the program should be transferred to the case manager.*

This change would accomplish the following: 1) eliminate one of the players from the already bewildering array of service providers; 2) give case managers more autonomy and flexibility in delivering individually tailored services; 3) improve the responsiveness of the system to changing client needs; 4) allow case managers additional opportunities to become acquainted with the client and her/his situation; and 5) make it easier to involve the client in the decision-making process, thus enhancing the client's independence and control of services.

Another program element that is a constant source of irritation and mistakes is communication. Our data show that in the CCSP, communication seems to break down from the very beginning—in the initial assessment of need. This breakdown seems to occur for two reasons. One reason is related to the client—either to her lack of knowledge about the program's ability to meet desired needs or to her hesitance to communicate the necessary information to the person making the assessment. Client reticence is based in feelings of powerlessness and in the client's need or desire to control information. It may result also from a learned wariness of government officials, especially those who are white, as most assessors are. Another barrier to communication is presented by the lack of skill of some assessors in putting the client at sufficient ease to communicate the needed information. Another is the assessor's lack of understanding of the client's situation and lifestyle, illustrated most clearly among our participants by the situation described above of the manager's unawareness of Mr. Jones and Mrs. Washington's relationship. Possession of such insight could add an intuitive dimension to the assessment interview that would produce better assessments. These problems could be addressed in part by better training of assessors in interviewing skills and in knowledge about their clients' culture and lifestyles in addition to their health statuses. We recommend:

12. *Communication should be improved among all participants in the care experience.*

Better communication is needed between assessors, case managers, RN supervisors, and aides. Although assessors outline clients' needs, it is the case manager who develops the care plan and orders the actual services. The typical communication between the two about a specific client is the annual assessment form. If the case manager, who visits every three months, observes a needed change, she can contact the assessor, who must make a special visit to re-evaluate the situation. The RN supervisor from the provider health agency is given the supervisory role in the ongoing care, and her communication with the case manager is rare. The typical communication between either the assessor or the case manager and the provider agency is with the agency liaison person, not a direct care provider. No communication exists between aides and either case managers or assessors unless they happen to visit simultaneously. Neither is communication between the RN supervisor and the aide a regular occurrence. It is therefore by necessity that the client herself often is the avenue of communication, where it exists, between all parts of the system. It is no wonder that confusion and misunderstandings occur. Problems of communication between clients and aides and clients and RN supervisors have been well-documented by these data. Regular care conferences between aides and RN's might solve some of these problems. Because of noted failures of communication and/or conflicts between informal caregivers and formal providers, increased efforts should be made, whenever possible, to involve family members and others providing supportive care.

Despite the problems of communication between aides and clients, their interface might be the most effective point in the system to make changes. Because of their greater similarity of race and status and, in many cases, of lifestyles, these clients feel a bond with their aides, at least compared with other actors in the system. The aides, too, are better equipped to understand and communicate with these black clients than most of their supervisors. The communication between aides and clients, and the resultant effectiveness of aide services, could be addressed in various ways. For one, aides could be better educated about the attitudes of their clients toward being helped, about how clients like to be helped, and how their own demeanor and method of providing care affects the way clients feel about themselves. They could be trained to be more intuitive in order to detect needs the client finds difficult to express. Most of this necessary education could and should come from the clients themselves. Aides must be given sufficient time to sit down with their clients and tell them what the aides are expected and willing to do, as Anne did with Ms. Worth. Clients then could tell the aides how they want the work done. Such communication would, of course, depend entirely on at least minimal continuity of the aide-client relationship.

The avenues of communication must be facilitated between the aides and the RN's as well so that aides can communicate the need for adjustments in the service plan. Aides must be made to feel that their opinions are valued, for they, along with the clients, are in reality the key to a successful care experience.

One final recommendation relates to the general reluctance of these clients to take action in response to situations they view as problematic. Improved avenues of communication throughout the system should at least partially address this problem. The clients' reluctance, however, often is motivated by an uneasy mixture of sympathy for the aides—typified by Mrs. Starr's not wanting to "break on my own color"—and fear of their reaction, as well as a pervasive feeling of powerlessness. In fact, because of their physical isolation from program supervisors and other authorities, home care clients are the most vulnerable of all long-term care recipients. We heard from our participants of two clear instances of abuse, only one of which was reported. One occurred when an aide slapped Mrs. Starr, and another involved an aide who borrowed money from Rev. Scott without repaying it. For these reasons, we recommend:

13. *An ombudsman-type program should be created to protect home care client and enhance their quality of care.*

We feel that extension of ombudsman-type protection and assistance to home care clients would offer additional impetus for clients to report problems and express their needs. Clients could be educated about their rights and encouraged to use them. By having someone totally unconnected to the program acting as their advocate, clients might be more forthcoming.

## IMPLICATIONS FOR RESEARCH

### For Theory and Knowledge

We have proposed that the value of independence is foremost in the minds and behavior of these African American elders as they navigate the waters of long-term care and evaluate their care. This value is composed of two interrelated elements—1) maintaining control over their lives and 2) maintaining an independent identity—and seems to gain importance as it becomes more elusive.

While independence sits squarely at the center of this complex long-term care situation, many other factors play key roles in shaping the daily lives of these participants and determining how the client defines quality care. Their race, their poverty, their lifestyles, their health status, and their health care practices all influence their needs for care. Their care needs, in turn, may determine what services they receive, but it is the type of services, the circumstances of their delivery, and the characteristics and behavior of those who provide them that determine whether the client feels well-served. These clients define quality of care in terms of the quality of the caring: if they feel comfortable with the caregiver, if they perceive she is genuinely concerned for their well-being, if they find the caregiver is willing to meet the client's special needs and preferences for how the care is given, and if the relationship affords an opportunity for meaningful social interaction, these clients will be quite satisfied with their care. Care may or may not be professionally adequate, and clients may or may not improve, but our data suggest they *will* be satisfied with the experience. On the other hand, the most technically proficient caregiver who fails to meet these criteria for quality, will be harshly judged by these clients.

A number of theoretical perspectives offer additional explanatory power for our data. Among these, we found exchange theory to fit best with the attitudes and behavior patterns of our participants. The basic premise of this theory—that in relationships of social exchange, participants act to maximize their benefits and reduce their costs—explains to a significant degree the strategies that these individuals use in their relationships with their caregivers. These strategies are designed to maximize the benefits derived from caregiving and to reduce the costs related to being dependent. The participants' intent in using them is to retain control of their lives and of the caregiving process to the extent possible, while striving to maintain an independent—and thus more valued and powerful—identity. When Mrs. Starr refuses to ask her aide to do her cooking or washing, she is reducing the costs associated with losing control over how these tasks are performed. She makes a rational decision based on her own cost/benefit analysis of her situation.

Applications of exchange theory in the field of aging [14-16] have suggested that the problems of dependency are based on the decline of resources found among older persons. Our data easily fit this explanation, since participants' remaining personal resources are key to the success of their caregiving relationships. With the decline of physical abilities and the continued scarcity of material and, for some, intellectual resources, these individuals use their psychological and spiritual resources and their interpersonal skills to achieve greater gain in exchange relationships. Social skills are most significant in negotiating and communicating with caregivers and also in managing one's identity to appear more independent—a strategy aimed ultimately at achieving increased power and control.

Because of the poverty of these participants and of many of their informal caregivers, the traditional altruism that often motivates people to help—out of the goodness of their hearts or for the sole reward of gratitude—is not operative in many of these exchanges. Poor people often cannot afford the luxury of altruism. In Mrs. Starr's experience, "People don't want thanks. They can't eat it. They can't spend it." We found that paying for help is an acceptable strategy among family and friends in situations of poverty where small, even token, monetary rewards are highly valued. It follows logically that a person who believes that offering money is a valid strategy to secure help from informal caregivers will use this same strategy to maximize rewards in relationships with formal caregivers, particularly when this behavior is supported by the belief that the desired task extracts significant costs from the caregiver.

In many instances, exchange behavior is a response to the social interactions incumbent in the caregiving process. In this light, symbolic interactionism [17] is a useful framework of orientation for our data. It is through social interactions that people define their social realities and sense of self. Through interpreting and evaluating the meanings of our interactions with others, we define each situation and use these definitions to guide our behavior. It is through interactions with others that these individuals define themselves and are defined by others as dependent and burdensome. These same interactions spawn their strategies to preserve their fading images of their former, more independent, selves. When Rev. Scott's niece complains that, because of other responsibilities, she is burdened and over-extended, he turns down her offer of Sunday dinner—for him, the least costly option. Mrs. Washington asks nothing more of the aide who frowned in response to her requests, and Mr. Avant's curt manner squelches Mrs. Little's requests, even for a drink of water. Others use money to counter-balance reluctant attitudes.

Identity theory [18] also emphasizes the human capacity to create a self-concept through social interactions. Those individuals who strive to be self-reliant and to manage their identities to portray greater independence are attempting to create for themselves an alternative role-identity to that of disabled, dependent, passive care-receiver. Although those clients who assume a significant role in the process of formal care are in part taking the least costly route (because no one else is assuming that role), they also are creating a valued role for themselves—care manager or care director—an active, important position.

The strategies these functionally disabled people use as they try to manage their lives, their care, and their identities all can be considered creative adaptations to their circumstances. Their actions can be explained under a number of organizing frameworks, all of which are valid and which sometimes operate simultaneously. It has been suggested that poor people are able to adapt better to the infirmities of old age and disability than more privileged persons, and, to the extent that an overriding value for independence is positively adaptive, these data support such a theory. The individuals portrayed here undoubtedly have developed creative adaptations to poverty over a lifetime of necessity, an experience that has prepared them for the declining physical, social, and material resources of old age. That is, a lifetime of having to maximize benefits and minimize costs in response to hardship is good training for surviving dependence. Perhaps the lengthier periods of disability experienced by Ms. Worth and Rev. Scott—Ms. Worth, in her definiton, since birth and Rev. Scott since his forties—offered them an even greater opportunity to prepare for their later dependency and to achieve greater successes in surviving it.

## For Method

It is clear to us that ethnography was an appropriate methodology for this study, since the aim was understanding an alternative view of reality—how these African American older persons, who are also poor and functionally disabled, experience their lives of dependency and interpret and use formal community-based services. Much of the information obtained was not learned at first asking, and much was not learned by asking at all. Sometimes it was necessary simply to let our informants talk about what was important to them. We found that in many cases being able to share their experiences was key. It was necessary to *be* at County Hospital to approach understanding of the patient's experiences. It was crucial to *observe* clients' interactions with their aides and informal caregivers to offer explanations of their behaviors. It was equally telling to *see* the still-full bottles of Mrs. Little's medicine and the trays containing Ms. Worth's home-delivered meals lying in her backyard, food only for the cat.

Also critical was having sufficient time to develop relationships of trust with these older people—a necessary prerequisite to be allowed to share a part of their lives. This was particularly true since the observer was white and middle class. With time, however, it was possible to overcome much of the racial divide and become a part of networks and experience caregiving relationships first-hand. Much of the information we wanted to find out is the kind most people are reluctant to share with anyone, especially a survey researcher, and for reasons of control, even their own family members. On one occasion the first author helped Mrs. Starr fill out a mailed survey from the home health agency that was serving her. Without that help, the questionnaire would have been ignored. In addition, she found the information required by some of the questions elusive and, on her own, would have omitted such items. The questions she did understand, she answered, with a smile, the way she thought was expected of her.

Equal to the element of trust in demanding a naturalistic approach, is the complexity of the situation. As emphasized in the presentation of data, the long-term care situation is composed of myriad factors, many of which interact with one another, and all subject to change. Knowing how these factors change and interact is fundamental to understanding the total situation [19]. Additionally, attitudinal factors often are key to how the situation is played out, affecting most of the behaviors involved. Attitudinal data also are often the most difficult to obtain from individuals, who, for a variety of reasons, are reluctant to express their true feelings.

## For Future Research

Much has been learned from this study about home care of older, disabled persons, but much remains unknown. An additional area of research that would help complete the picture would involve the viewpoints of the aides themselves, as well as those of RN supervisors, case managers, assessors, and those at the planning level. Although some data from the aides' point of view were gathered during this research, much remains to be learned. Of particular interest would be how the different types of providers view their own jobs, the jobs of others, their clients, their clients' roles, and the degree to which these varying viewpoints coincide. Such information could be used in furthering understanding and communication throughout the system. Intensive interviewing and participant observation of caregivers as they act out their roles would be an appropriate methodology.

Other components of community-based care, such as adult day rehabilitation centers and residential care facilities, offer fruitful areas of exploration. Information about how services are experienced and received in both settings is needed. For the same reasons considered in this research, a naturalistic approach would be essential to capture the behaviors and meanings necessary for understanding.

While no broad generalizations can be drawn from this study, the insights presented here can be applied in similar home care situations where care recipients are poor, elderly, and black. Where the total picture is not readily applicable, meanings can be drawn from different parts of the data and applied in a variety of situations related to dependency, long-term care, poverty, and health care. Thus, naturalistic researchers speak of transferability, rather than generalizability.

## CONCLUDING THOUGHTS

In addition to being poor and disabled, each of these African American elders has another trait in common—the will to keep trying. Some may grieve and some may not accomplish much, but nobody has given up. This trait is sometimes their best defense.

Many of their problems are related to being black and poor. For these individuals, growing up as they did in a Jim Crow society and being both subjects and objects of a lifelong and intense racial consciousness, race has undoubtedly been a defining fact of life. To a large extent, it determined their life chances by denying them equal educational and occupational opportunities. While some of our participants were more race conscious than others, race continues for all as a filter through which every facet of life and behavior of others is viewed, assayed, and evaluated. We strongly believe the physical and emotional similarities of dependency coupled with the seemingly universal commitment to independence outweigh the cultural differences between the races. Yet, the importance of being old, poor, sick, *and* black should not be minimized.

Being poor for most of their lives has affected these individuals' present economic situations, their homes, their neighborhoods, and their character. Poverty has affected their education levels, employment histories, and current levels of Social Security benefits. It has had a major impact on their health statuses and on their attitudes and practices related to health care. Poverty also has influenced the economic situation of their informal caregivers. This life of poverty has determined many of their needs for formal long-term care services.

It is because of poverty that these participants are eligible for the Community Care Services Program—the program that pays for most of their formal long-term care services. For the most part, they are extremely grateful for these services, and the services meet many basic needs. Doubtless, some of these needs would go unmet without these services, and probably one or two persons even would be institutionalized. Social worlds are expanded by visits from formal caregivers, and some clients even develop close emotional ties with their aides. The burdens of some family caregivers are considerably lightened. Certainly, these services are beneficial to the clients who receive them; and without doubt, the cry of these dependent persons to remain in their own homes is loud and clear. The need for more programs providing community-based care, both now and in the future, is also clear.

We have seen that some of these clients still have needs for care that remain after the last aide has left and friends and family members have all gone home. Some of these unmet needs are related to flaws in the program, which have been pointed out, and some suggestions have been made for program improvements. While improvements are certainly possible and could benefit clients in important ways, many needs of these older disabled persons are more basic—those related to their life chances and poverty. Because these problems are more intransigent and their solutions more costly, they are met with resistance by lawmakers. But these issues also must be addressed—not just for old, disabled African Americans, but for children and for all others with similar problems who, one day, will be old, too.

## REFERENCES

1. N. L . Chappell, Home Care Research: What Does It Tell Us? *The Gerontologist, 34*:1, pp. 116-120, 1994.
2. N. N. Eustis, R. A. Kane, and L. R. Fischer, Home Care Quality and the Home Care Worker: Beyond Quality Assurance as Usual, *The Gerontologist, 33*:1, pp. 64-73, 1993.
3. C. P. Sabatino, Client-Rights Regulations and the Autonomy of Home-Care Consumers, *Generations, XIV:*Supplement, pp. 21-24, 1990.
4. N. N. Dubler, Autonomy and Accommodation: Mediating Individual Choice in the Home Setting, *Generations, XIV*: Supplement, pp. 29-31, 1990.
5. M. B. Kapp, Home Care Client-Centered Systems: Consumer Choice vs. Protection, *Generations, XIV:* Supplement, pp. 33-35, 1990.
6. C. H. Hennessy, Autonomy and Risk: The Role of Client Wishes in Community-Based Long-Term Care, *The Gerontologist, 29*:5, pp. 633-639, 1989.
7. M. Weber, *From Max Weber: Essays in Sociology,* H. Gerth and C. W. Mills (eds. and trans.), Oxford University Press, New York, 1958.
8. M. Cantor and E. Chichin, *Stress and Strain Among Home Care Workers of the Frail Elderly,* Brookdale Research Institute on Aging, Third Age Center, Fordham University, New York, 1990.
9. N. N. Eustis and L. R. Fischer, Relationships Between Home Care Clients and Their Workers: Implications for Quality of Care, *The Gerontologist, 31*:4, pp. 447-456, 1991.

10. M. MacAdam, Home Care Reimbursement and Effects on Personnel, *The Gerontologist, 33*:1, 55-63, 1993.
11. P. Feldman, Work Life Improvements for Home Care Workers: Impact and Feasibility, *The Gerontologist, 33*:1, pp. 47-54, 1993.
12. J. Rothman, A Model of Case Management: Toward Empirically Based Practice, *Social Work, 36*, pp. 520-527, 1991.
13. J. A. Altholz and M. L. Duggar, *Mobilizing Community Resources: A Case Management Perspective*, Georgia Department of Human Resources, Office of Aging, 1985.
14. J. Dowd, Aging as Exchange: A Preface to Theory, *Journal of Gerontology, 30*, pp. 584-594, 1975.
15. S. Matthews, *The Social World of Old Women: Management of Self-Identity*, Sage Publications, Inc., Beverly Hills, California, 1979.
16. K. A. Roberto, Equity in Friendships, in *Older Adult Friendships*, R. G. Adams and R. Blieszner (eds.), Sage Publications, Inc., Newbury Park, California, pp. 147-165, 1989.
17. R. H. Turner, Unanswered Questions in the Convergence between Structuralist and Interactionist, in *Micro-Theory*, H. J. Helle and S. N. Eisenstadt (eds.), Volume 2, Sage Publications, Inc., London, 1985.
18. S. Stryker and R. Serpe, Commitment, Identity Salience, and Role Behavior: Theory and Research Example, in *Personality, Roles, and Social Behavior*, W. Ickes and E. S. Knowles (eds.), Springer-Verlag, New York, pp. 199-218, 1982.
19. C. H. Hennessy and M. Hennessy, Community-Based Long-Term Care for the Elderly: Evaluation Practice Reconsidered, *Medical Care Review, 47*:2, pp. 221-259, 1990.

# Epilogue

## ELOISE LITTLE

Mrs. Little spent her last Christmas in County Hospital. The deterioration of her body had continued without pause, and she complained of an overwhelming tiredness. When she entered the hospital in mid-December, her half-sisters initiated plans for nursing placement. As if to exert a final measure of control, on January 22, 1991, Mrs. Little passed away. Fourteen people attended her funeral. Among them were Mr. Avant, Miss Fannie, and Rosa Mae. Mrs. Little's house has the look of abandonment, but Mr. Avant remains a loyal tenant. He looks out now for Miss Fannie, who is herself homebound, making daily trips to lock and unlock her door, as he once did for Mrs. Little.

## RUBY WASHINGTON

Ruby Washington died in the summer of 1991, soon after her eighty-sixth birthday. She too spent her last days in County Hospital. Her heart just "gave out," Mr. Jones said. The neighborhood church she loved to attend was filled with church members, family, and friends come to bid her farewell.

## LUCY OLIVER

In the summer of 1991, Lucy Oliver and her husband moved from the housing project where they had resided their entire married life to a highrise for the elderly in the suburbs. While highrise life held no appeal for either one, they succumbed to family pleas to flee the neighborhood violence. Before Mrs. Oliver could become acclimated to her new home, she suffered a second and fatal stroke. She was seventy-six years old.

## SALLY FINCH

Sally Finch maintained a life of seclusion in her highrise apartment until she met with an unexpected death on March 30, 1992. She was eighty-one years of age. Her niece reported that apparently she fell while getting into bed and became wedged between the bed and dresser. The security guard at the highrise found her dead the next morning. The modest group of family and friends who gathered for her funeral included Doright, her loyal helper.

## GERALDINE STARR

Geraldine Starr died January 21, 1994, in the intensive care unit at County Hospital. She would have been eighty years old on her next birthday, Valentine's Day. Because she willed her body to science, she had no burial. Not even a notice in the paper marked her passing.

Mrs. Starr's decline was imperceptible at first. During the renovation of her highrise, she had to vacate the apartment she had occupied for ten years. The move was stressful, and she never quite grew accustomed to her new environment. She became confused about her medications and often was groggy, sleeping for hours upright in her chair. One night, while on her way to the bathroom, she fell and lost consciousness. Her aide found her the next morning lying on the floor, awake but disoriented. Unfamiliar with Mrs. Starr's health care arrangements, the aide instructed the emergency technician to take Mrs. Starr to County Memorial instead of the private hospital where Dr. Moore, her regular physician, admitted her patients. Try though she might, Mrs. Starr was never able to maneuver a transfer, and, instead, was persuaded to give up her apartment and enter a nursing home.

At the nursing home Mrs. Starr's health improved. She reverted to her alert and feisty self, complaining regularly about "the way they put the crazy ones in with the ones that still got good sense," about her confused roommate—who accused her of "stealing her things"—and about the "horse slop" she was served for meals. Despite her incessant grumbling, Mrs. Starr was popular with the staff. They loved her prickly ways and sometimes supplied her with extra food.

From the first day, however, Mrs. Starr was steadfast in her pursuit of freedom and achieved success when Lenore, the telephone operator at her bank, offered her a place in her home. Lenore had cared for people from time to time and needed the extra income. She gave Mrs. Starr her own room with a double bed. Lenore's daughter, who was unemployed, usually stayed at home during the day and prepared Mrs. Starr's meals and administered her medications. Lenore's toy poodle often napped on Mrs. Starr's bed.

Although content at first in Lenore's home, Mrs. Starr soon began to express dissatisfaction and anxiety. The daughter scared her sometimes, acted like she "took dope." She frequently had a man with her. Still Mrs. Starr was adamant in her refusal to return to the nursing home, proclaiming she would "rather be dead." Only six weeks after her move to Lenore's, she was admitted to the intensive care unit at County Hospital. Her doctors said she had suffered another stroke and held no hope for her recovery. Mrs. Starr once said, "Don't give up till the war is over." This was her final battle.

## VIOLA WORTH

Viola Worth is "still a truckin'," but she has slowed down a bit. Unrelenting pain in her right hip—the one that was replaced over four years ago—drove her back to the hospital for additional surgery in mid-January. The surgery was long, over ten hours, but appeared successful. Transferred to a rehabilitation hospital a week after surgery, she soon found the road to recovery blocked. After only a few days of therapy, the hip prosthesis slipped out of place, resulting in a second surgery. Next followed another week in the hospital and then a lengthy stint at the rehabilitation center. At this point Ms. Worth announced, "If I don't even live after I leave here, I don't care. I want to go *home!*"

Five months have elapsed since the surgery, and Ms. Worth spends much of her time in bed, still unable to walk without assistance. Undaunted in spirit, she gets by with help from her play children and daily home health aide services. A student from Africa, whom she took in as a roomer, stays with her at night.

While Ms. Worth's caregiving arrangements mirror those she has had in the past, some of the players have changed. Her god-daughter, Maxine, is no longer counted among her adopted children, a rift precipitated by Maxine's appropriation of Ms. Worth's money to pay her own bills. Ms. Worth was hurt when Maxine let her down but soon substituted Barbara as number one play daughter. Her beloved aide, Anne, long since transferred, has been succeeded by an assortment of aides. One, Ms. Worth discharged because of her recalcitrant attitude. The Foster Grandparents Program has furnished additional helpers, and a home repair organization has brightened her house, both inside and out.

While Ms. Worth admits she never has had "to be quiet" like she must now, she still is proud she can "do pretty good" and is ever-optimistic that God "will open another door."

## REV. JOSEPH SCOTT

Rev. Scott has been back in the hospital three times for additional skin graft surgery, each without success. When his regular surgeon started "talking amputation," he found a new one. Results, however, have been no better. The graft from his most recent surgery refuses to heal, and during this last hospital stay, a fracture was discovered in his "good" leg.

Despite some "rough" days, Rev. Scott is "managing pretty good." He has a hospital bed, and his home-delivered services have been increased. A home health aide visits on Mondays and Wednesdays, and his personal support aide (PSA) comes five days per week. It means a lot that his new PSA likes to cook, but he misses his case manager, who left the program after being with him over five years. While Deacon Pate has had to abandon his caregiving role due to his own failing health and the competing demands of his wife, Rev. Scott's niece and brother continue to fill in when needed. During a recent two-month period when he was unable to get into bed by himself, they alternated coming to his house each evening.

In 1992, with the help of his family, Rev. Scott published a collection of sermons he either delivered during his years of preaching or hopes still to deliver someday. A quote from his book, embodies the strong faith that is his mainstay: "Prayer is one of the surest means of attaining a higher spirituality as well as one of the strongest staffs upon which to lean when weak or troubled."

# Bibliography

Abel, E. K., Daughters Caring for Elderly Parents, *The Home Care Experience*, J. F. Gubrium and A. Sankar (eds.), Sage Publications, Inc., Newbury Park, California, 1990.

Abeles, R. P., H. G. Gift, and M. G. Ory (eds.), *Aging and Quality of Life: Charting New Territories in Behavioral Science Research*, Springer Publishing Company, New York, 1994.

Administration on Aging, Infrastructure of Home and Community Based Services for Functionally Impaired Elderly, *State Source Book*, U.S. Department of Health and Human Services, 1994.

Agency for Health Care Policy and Research, *Nonreimbursed Home Health Care: Beyond the Bills*, Washington, D.C., 1990.

Allan, G. A. and R. G. Adams, Aging and the Structure of Friendship, *Older Adult Friendships*, R. G. Adams and R. Blieszner (eds.), Sage Publications, Inc., Newbury Park, California, pp. 45-64, 1989.

Allen, K. R. and V. Chin-Sang, A Lifetime of Work: The Context and Meanings of Leisure for Aging Black Women, *The Gerontologist, 30*:1, pp. 734-740, 1990.

Altholz, J. A. and M. L. Duggar, *Mobilizing Community Resources: A Case Management Perspective*, Georgia Department of Human Resources, Office of Aging, 1985.

American Association of Retired Persons, *Building a Better Health Care System: America's Challenge of the 1990s*, Washington, D. C., 1990.

American Association of Retired Persons and Administration on Aging, *A Profile of Older Americans: 1993*, Washington, D.C., 1993.

American Health Care Association, *A Proposal for Long Term Care Financing Reform*, Washington, D.C., 1993.

Applebaum, R. and J. Christian, Using Case Management to Monitor Community-based Long-term Care, *QRB, 14*, pp. 227-231, 1988.

Aschenbrenner, J., *Lifelines: Black Families in Chicago*, Holt, Rinehart, and Winston, New York, 1975.

Barer, B. M., The Relationship Between Homebound Older People and Their Home Care Worker, *Journal of Gerontological Social Work, 19*, pp. 129-147, 1992.

Barker, J. C. and L. S. Mitteness, Invisible Caregivers in the Spotlight: Non-kin Caregivers of Frail Older Adults, *The Home Care Experience*, J. F. Gubrium and A. Sankar (eds.), Sage Publications, Inc., Newbury Park, California, 1990.

Berwick, D. and M. Knapp, Theory and Practice for Measuring Health Care Quality, *Health Care Financing Review, 9*:Supplement, pp. 49-55, 1987.

Bloom, S. W. and R. Wilson, Patient-Practitioner Relationships, *Handbook of Medical Sociology*, H. E. Freeman, S. Levine, and L. G. Reeder (eds.), Prentice-Hall, Englewood Cliffs, New Jersey, pp. 275-296, 1972.

Branch, L. G. and A. M. Jette, Elders' Use of Informal Long-term Care Assistance, *The Gerontologist, 23*, pp. 51-56, 1983.

Braun, K. and C. Rose, The Hawaii Geriatric Foster Care Experiment: Impact Evaluation and Cost Analysis, *The Gerontologist, 26*, pp. 515-524, 1986.

Braun, K. L., L. Goto, and A. Lenzer, Patient Age and Satisfaction with Home Care, *Home Health Care Services Quarterly, 8*, pp. 79-96, 1987.

Brody, E., "Women in the Middle" and Family Help to Older People, *The Gerontologist, 21*, pp. 471-480, 1981.

Brody, S. J., W. Poulshock, and C. F. Musciocchi, The Family Caring Unit: A Major Consideration in the Long-term Support System, *The Gerontologist, 18*, pp. 556-561, 1978.

Brubaker, T. H. (ed.), *Family Relations in Later Life*, Sage Publications, Inc., Beverly Hills, California, 1983.

Cantor, M., Life Space and the Social Support System of the Inner City Elderly of New York, *The Gerontologist, 15*, pp. 23-27, 1975.

Cantor, M., Neighbors and Friends: An Overlooked Resource in Informal Support Systems, *Research on Aging, 1*:4, pp. 434-463, 1979.

Cantor, M., *Caring for the Frail Elderly: Impact on Family, Friends and Neighbors*, Paper presented at 33rd Annual Meeting of The Gerontological Society of America, San Diego, California, 1980.

Cantor, M., Strain Among Caregivers: A Study of Experience in the United States, *The Gerontologist, 23*, pp. 597-604, 1983.

Cantor, M., Families: A Basic Source of Long-term Care for the Elderly, *Aging, 349*, pp. 8-13, 1985.

Cantor, M. and E. Chichin, *Stress and Strain Among Home Care Workers of the Frail Elderly*, Brookdale Research Institute on Aging, Third Age Center, Fordham University, New York, 1990.

Cantor, M. and M. Mayer, Factors in Differential Utilization of Services by Urban Elderly, *Journal of Gerontological Social Work, 1*:1, pp. 47-62, 1978.

Carlsson-Agren, M., S. Berg, and C. G. Wenestam, Daily Life of the Oldest Old, *Journal of Sociology & Social Welfare, 19*:2, pp. 109-124, 1992.

Challis, D. and C. Davies, Home Care of the Frail Elderly in the United Kingdom: Matching Resources to Needs, *Home Health Care Services Quarterly, 5*, pp. 89-109, 1985.

Chappell, N. L., Informal Support Networks Among the Elderly, *Research on Aging, 5*:1, pp. 77-99, 1983.

Chappell, N. L., Home Care Research: What Does It Tell Us?, *The Gerontologist, 34*:1, pp. 116-120, 1994.

Chatters, L. M., R. J. Jackson, and J. S. Jackson, Aged Blacks' Choices for an Informal Helper Network, *Journal of Gerontology, 41*:1, pp. 94-100, 1986.

Choi, N. G., Patterns and Determinants of Social Service Utilization: Comparison of the Childless Elderly and Elderly Parents Living with or Apart from their Children, *The Gerontologist, 34*:3, pp. 353-362, 1994.

Chubon, S. J., Personal Descriptions of Compliance by Rural Southern Blacks, *Journal of Compliance in Health Care, 4*:1, pp. 23-38, 1989.

Cohen, C. and J. Sokolovsky, Social Engagement versus Isolation: The Case of the Aged in SRO Hotels, *The Gerontologist, 20*, pp. 36-40, 1980.

Collopy, B., Autonomy in Long Term Care: Some Crucial Distinctions, *The Gerontologist, 28*, pp. 10-17, Supplement 1988.

Collopy, B. J., Ethical Dimensions of Autonomy in Long-Term Care, *Generations, XIV*:Supplement, pp. 9-12, 1990.

Corbin, J. M. and A. Strauss, Making Arrangements: The Key to Home Care, *The Home Care Experience*, J. Gubrium and A. Sankar (eds.), Sage Publications, Inc., Newbury Park, California, pp. 59-74, 1990.

Crohan, S. E. and T. C. Antonucci, Friends as a Source of Social Support in Old Age, *Older Adult Friendships*, R. G. Adams and R. Blieszner (eds.), Sage Publications, Inc., Newbury Park, California, pp. 129-146, 1989.

Crossman, L., C. London, and C. Barry, Older Women Caring for Disabled Spouses: A Model for Supportive Services, *The Gerontologist, 21*, pp. 464-470, 1981.

Czaja, S. J., R. A. Weber, and S. N. Nair, A Human Factor Analysis of ADL Activities: A Capability Demand Approach, *Journal of Gerontology, 48*, pp. 44-50, 1993.

DeFriese, G. H., T. R. Konrad, A. Woomert, J. K. Norburn, and S. Bernard, Self-Care and Quality of Life in Old Age, *Aging and Quality of Life: Charting New Territories in Behavorial Science Research*, R. P. Abeles, H. G. Gift, and M. G. Ory (eds.), Springer Publishing Company, New York, 1994.

Deimling, G. T. and W. S. Poulshock, Families Caring for Elders in Residence: Issues in the Measurement of Burden, *Journal of Gerontology, 39*, pp. 230-234, 1984.

Doty, P., K. Liu, and J. Wiener, An Overview of Long-Term Care, *Health Care Financing Review, 6*, pp. 69-78, 1985.

Dougherty, M. C., *Becoming a Woman in Rural Black Culture*, Holt, Rinehart and Winston, New York, 1978.

Dowd, J., Aging as Exchange: A Preface to Theory, *Journal of Gerontology, 30*, pp. 584-594, 1975.

Dowd, J., Exchange Rates and Old People, *Journal of Gerontology, 35*, pp. 596-602, 1980.

Dowd, J., *Stratification Among the Aged*, Wadsworth Publishing Company, California, 1980.

Dressel, P. L., Gender, Race and Class in Later Life, *The Gerontologist, 28*:2, pp. 177-180, 1988.

Dressel, P. L., *The Service Trap*, Charles C. Thomas, Publishers, Springfield, Illinois, 1984.

Dubler, N. N., Autonomy and Accommodation: Mediating Individual Choice in the Home Setting, *Generations, XIV*:Supplement, pp. 29-31, 1990.

Emerson, R. M., *Contemporary Field Research: A Collection of Readings*, Waveland Press, Prospect Heights, Illinois, 1983.

Eustis, N. N. and L. R. Fischer, Relationships Between Home Care Clients and Their Workers: Implications for Quality of Care, *The Gerontologist, 31*:4, pp. 447-456, 1991.

Eustis, N. N., R. A. Kane, and L. R. Fischer, Home Care Quality and the Home Care Worker: Beyond Quality Assurance as Usual, *The Gerontologist, 33*:1, pp. 64-73, 1993.

Feldman, P., Work Life Improvements for Home Care Workers: Impact and Feasibility, *The Gerontologist, 33*:1, pp. 47-54, 1993.

Fischer, L. R., L. Rogne, and N. N. Eustis, Support Systems for the Familyless Elderly: Care Without Commitment, in *The Home Care Experience*, J. F. Gubrium and A. Sankar (eds.), Sage Publications, Inc., Newbury Park, California, 1990.

Fries, J. F. and J. F. Crapo, The Elimination of Premature Disease, in *Wellness and Health Promotion for the Elderly*, K. Dychtwald (ed.), Aspen Systems Corporation, Rockville, Maryland, pp. 19-37, 1986.

Fry, C., *Aging in Culture and Society: Comparative Viewpoints and Strategies*, J. R. Bergin, Brooklyn, 1980.

Geertz, C., Thick Description: Toward an Interpretative Theory of Culture, in *Contemporary Field Research*, R. M. Emerson (ed.), Waveland Press, Prospect Heights, Illinois, 1983.

Gibson, R. C. and J. S. Jackson, The Health, Physical Functioning, and Informal Supports of the Black Elderly, *The Milbank Quarterly, 65*, pp. 421-454, 1987.

Glaser, B. and A. Strauss, *The Discovery of Grounded Theory: Strategies for Qualitative Research*, Aldine, Chicago, 1967.

Goffman, E., *The Presentation of Self in Everyday Life*, Anchor Books, New York, 1959.

Goffman, E., *Stigma: Notes on Management of Spoiled Identity*, Prentice Hall, Englewood Cliffs, New Jersey, 1963.

Gold, D. T., Late-life Sibling Relationships: Does Race Affect Typological Distribution? *The Gerontologist, 30*:6, pp. 741-748, 1990.

Goodman, C. C., Natural Helping Among Older Adults, *The Gerontologist, 24*, pp. 138-143, 1984.

Gubrium, J., *Living and Dying at Murray Manor*, St. Martin's, New York, 1975.

Gubrium, J., *The Mosaic of Care*, Springer Publishing Company, New York, 1991.

Gubrium, J. F. and A. Sankar (eds.), *The Home Care Experience*, Sage Publications, Inc., Newbury Park, California, 1990.

Hannerz, U., *Soulside: Inquiries into Ghetto Culture and Community*, Columbia University Press, New York, 1969.

Harrington, C., Quality, Access and Costs: Public Policy and Home Health Care, *Nursing Outlook, 36*, pp. 164-166, 1988.

Harrington, C. and L. A. Grant, The Delivery, Regulation, and Politics of Home Care: A California Case Study, *The Gerontologist, 30*:4, pp. 451-461, 1990.

Haskins, K. B., J. Capitman, F. Colligen, B. Degraaf, and C. Yordi, *Evaluation of Community Long-term Care Demonstration Projects: Extramural Report*, Health Care Financing Administration, Baltimore, 1987.

Hatch, L. R., Informal Support Patterns of Older African-American and White Women, *Research on Aging, 13*:2, pp. 144-170, 1991.

Hays, W. C. and C. H. Mindel, Extended Kinship Relations in Black and White Families, *Journal of Marriage and the Family, 35*, pp. 51-57, 1973.

Health Care Financing Administration, Bureau of Data Management and Strategy, 1993 HCFA Statistics, HCFA Pub. No. 03341, June 1993.

Hennessy, C. H., Autonomy and Risk: The Role of Client Wishes in Community-Based Long-Term Care, *The Gerontologist, 29*, pp. 633-639, 1989.

Hennessy, C. H. and M. Hennessy, Community-Based Long-Term Care for the Elderly: Evaluation Practice Reconsidered, *Medical Care Review, 47*:2, pp. 221-259, 1990.

Hickey, T., *Health and Aging*, Brooks Cole, Monterey, California, 1980.

Hill, A. C. and F. Jaffe, Negro Fertility and Family Size Preferences: Implications for Programming of Health and Social Services, in *The Black Family: Essays and Studies*, R. Staples (ed.), Wadsworth Publishing Company, Belmont, California, 1971.

Hill, R. B., *The Strength of Black Families*, Emerson Hall, New York, 1974.

Hochschild, A. *The Unexpected Community*, Prentice Hall, Englewood Cliffs, New Jersey, 1973.

Hofland, B. F., Why a Special Focus on Autonomy?, *Generations, XIV*:Supplement, pp. 5-8, 1990.

Hulling, W. E., Evolving Family Roles for the Black Elderly, *Aging, 287*, pp. 21-27, 1978.

Jackson, J. J., *Minorities and Aging*, Wadsworth Publishing Co., Belmont, California, 1980.

Jackson, J. J., "But What I Really Said Was": On Categorical Differences of Older Black Women, *Journal of Minority Aging, 5*, pp. 279-285, 1980.

Jackson, J. J., Race, National Origin, Ethnicity and Aging, in *Handbook of Aging and the Social Sciences*, R. H. Binstock and E. Shanas (eds.) (2nd Edition), Van Nostrand Reinhold, New York, pp. 264-303, 1985.

Jackson, J. J. and C. Perry, Physical Health Conditions of Middle-Aged and Aged Blacks, in *Aging and Health: Perspectives on Race, Ethnicity and Class*, K. Markides (ed.), Sage Publications, Inc., Newbury Park, California, pp. 111-176, 1989.

James, A., W. L. James, and H. L. Smith, Reciprocity as a Coping Strategy of the Elderly: A Rural Irish Perspective, *The Gerontologist, 24*, pp. 483-489, 1984.

James, W., The Self, in *The Principles of Psychology*, Henry Holt, New York, pp. 292-299, 1896.

Jette, A. M., L. G. Branch, L. A. Sleeper, H. Feldman, and L. M. Sullivan, High-risk Profiles for Nursing Home Admission, *The Gerontologist, 32*:5, pp. 635-640, 1992.

Johnson, C. L., Dyadic Family Relations and Social Support, *The Gerontologist, 23*, pp. 377-383, 1983.

Johnson, C. L. and B. Barer, Families and Networks Among Older Inner-City Blacks, *The Gerontologist, 30*, pp. 726-733, 1990.

Johnson, C. L. and D. J. Catalano, Childless Elderly and Their Family Supports, *The Gerontologist, 2*, pp. 610-618, 1981.

Johnson, C. L. and D. J. Catalano, A Longitudinal Study of Family Supports to Impaired Elderly, *The Gerontologist, 23*, pp. 612-618, 1983.

Johnson, C. L. and L. E. Troll, Constraints and Facilitators to Friendships in Late Late Life, *The Gerontologist, 34*:1, pp. 79-87, 1994.

Jonas, K., Factors in the Development of Community among Elderly Persons in Age-Segregated Housing: Relationships Between Involvement in Friendship Roles with the Community and External Social Roles, *Anthropological Quarterly, 52*, pp. 29-38, 1979.

Jonas, K. and E. Wellin, Dependency and Reciprocity: Home Health Aid in an Elderly Population, in *Aging in Culture and Society: Comparative Viewpoints and Strategies*, C. Fry (ed.), J. F. Bergin, Brooklyn, 1980.

Kalish, R., Of Children and Grandfathers: A Speculative Essay on Dependence, *The Gerontologist, 7*, pp. 65-79, 1967.

Kapp, M. B., Home Care Client-Centered Systems: Consumer Choice vs. Protection, *Generations, XIV*:Supplement, pp. 33-35, 1990.

Kaufman, S., *The Ageless Self: Sources of Meaning in Late Life*, The University of Wisconsin Press, Madison, Wisconsin, 1986.

Keith, J., *Old People As People: Social and Cultural Influences on Aging and Old Age*, Little, Brown, Boston, 1982.

Kemper, P., R. Brown, G. Carcagno, R. Applebaum, J. Christianson, W. Carson, S. Dunstan, T. Granneman, M. Harrigan, N. Holden, R. Phillips, J. Schore, C. Thornton, J. D. Wooldridge, and F. Skidmore, *The Evaluation of the National Long-term Care Demonstrations Final Report*, Mathematica Policy Research, Inc., Princeton, New Jersey, 1986.

Kendig, H. and D. Rowland, Family Support of the Australian Aged: Comparison with the United States, *The Gerontologist, 23*, pp. 643-649, 1983.

Kidder, T., *Old Friends*, Houghton-Mifflin Co., New York, 1993.

Lawton, M. P. and L. Nahemow, Ecology and the Aging Process, in *The Psychology of Adult Development and Aging*, C. Eisdorfer and M. P. Lawton (eds.), American Psychological Association, Washington, D.C., pp. 619-674, 1973.

Letsch, S. W., H. C. Lazenby, K. R. Levit, and C. A. Cowan, National Health Expenditures, 1991, *Health Care Financing Review, 14*:2, pp. 1-30, 1992.

Levitan, T. E., Deviants As Active Participants in the Labeling Process: The Visibly Handicapped, *Social Problems, 22*, pp. 548-557, 1975.

Levkoff, S. E., P. D. Cleary, T. Wetle, and R. W. Besdine, Illness Behavior in the Aged: Implications for Clinicians, *Journal of the American Geriatrics Society, 36*, pp. 622-629, 1988.

Liebow, E., *Tally's Corner: A Study of Negro Streetcorner Men*, Little, Brown, Boston, 1967.

Linn, M. and B. Linn, Qualities of Institutional Care that Affect Outcome, *Aged Care and Services Review, 2*, pp. 1-13, 1980.

Lockery, S. A., Family and Social Supports: Caregiving Among Racial and Ethnic Minority Elders, *Generations, XV*:1, pp. 58-62, 1991.

Lofland, J. and L. H. Lofland, *Analyzing Social Settings: A Guide to Qualitative Observation and Analysis* (2nd Edition), Wadsworth Publishing Co., Belmont, California, 1984.

Longino, Jr., C. F., G. Warheit, and J. A. Green, Class, Aging and Health, in *Aging and Health: Perspectives on Race, Ethnicity and Class*, K. Markides (ed.), Sage Publications, Inc., Newbury Park, California, pp. 79-110, 1989.

Lustbader, W., *Counting on Kindness: The Dilemmas of Dependency*, The Free Press, New York, 1991.

MacAdam, M., Home Care Reimbursement and Effects on Personnel, *The Gerontologist, 33*:1, pp. 55-63, 1993.

MacRae, H., Fictive Kin as a Component of the Social Networks of Older People, *Research on Aging, 14*:2, pp. 226-247, 1992.

Manton, K. G., L. S. Corder, and E. Stallard, Estimates of Change in Chronic Disability and Institutional Incidence and Prevalence Rates in the U.S. Elderly Population from the 1982, 1984, and 1989 National Long Term Care Survey, *Journal of Gerontology: Social Sciences, 48*:4, pp. S153-S166, 1993.

Manuel, R. C. and M. L. Berk, A Look at Similarities and Differences in Older Minority Populations, *Aging, 339*, pp. 21-29, 1983.

Markides, K., *Aging and Health: Perspectives on Race, Ethnicity and Class*, Sage Publications, Inc., Newbury Park, California, 1989.

Maslach, C., The Client Role in Staff Burnout, *Journal of Social Issues, 34*, pp. 111-124, 1978.

Matthews, S., *The Social World of Old Women: Management of Self-Identity*, Sage Publications, Inc., Beverly Hills, California, 1979.

McCann, B., The JCAH Home Care Project, *QRB, 16*, pp. 191-193, 1986.

McCann, J., Long-term Home Care for the Elderly: Perceptions of Nurses, Physicians, and Primary Caregivers, *QRB, 18*, pp. 66-74, 1988.

Mechanic, D., Illness Behavior: An Overview, in *Illness Behavior: A Multidisciplinary Model*, S. McHugh and T. M. Vallis (eds.), Plenum, New York, pp. 101-108, 1986.

Merrimam, S. B., *Case Study Research in Education: A Qualitative Approach*, Jossey-Bass Publishers, San Francisco, 1988.

Merton, R. K., Insiders and Outsiders: A Chapter in the Sociology of Knowledge, in *A History of Sociological Analysis*, T. Bottomore and R. Nisbet (eds.), Basic Books, New York, pp. 9-46, 1978.

Mitchell, J. and J. C. Register, An Exploration of Family Interaction with the Elderly by Race, Socioeconomic Status and Residence, *The Gerontologist, 24*, pp. 48-54, 1984.

Montgomery, R. and K. Kosloski, A Longitudinal Analysis of Nursing Home Placement for Dependent Elders Cared For By Spouses Versus Adult Children, *Journal of Gerontology: Social Sciences, 49*, pp. S62-S74, 1994.

Morris, J. and S. Sherwood, Informal Support Resources for Vulnerable Elderly Persons: Can They Be Counted On, Why Do They Work? *International Journal of Aging and Human Development, 18*, pp. 81-98, 1984.

Mumma, N., Quality and Cost Control of Home Care Services Through Coordinated Funding, *QRB, 17*, pp. 271-278, 1987.

Murtaugh, C. M., P. Kemper, and B. C. Spillman, The Risk of Nursing Home Use in Later Life, *Medical Care, 28*:10, pp. 952-962, 1990.

Mutran, E., Intergenerational Family Support Among Blacks and Whites: Response to Culture or to Socioeconomic Differences, *Journal of Gerontology, 40*:3, pp. 382-389, 1985.

Myerhoff, B., *Number Our Days*, Simon & Schuster, New York, 1978.

National Citizens' Coalition for Nursing Home Reform, *A Consumer Perspective on Quality of Care: The Residents' Point of View*, Washington, D.C., 1985.

Ness, K. M., The Sick Role of the Elderly, in *Psychosocial Nursing Care of the Aged*, I. M. Burnside (ed.), McGraw-Hill, New York, 1980.

O'Brien, M., *Anatomy of a Nursing Home: A View of Residential Life*, National Health Publishing, Owings Mills, Maryland, 1989.

O'Conner, P., Same-Gender and Cross-Gender Friendships Among the Frail Elderly, *The Gerontologist, 33*, pp. 24-30, 1993.

Petchers, M. K. and S. Milligan, Access to Health Care in a Black Urban Population, *The Gerontologist, 28*:2, pp. 213-217, 1988.

Roberson, M. H. B., The Meaning of Compliance: Patient Perspectives, *Qualitative Health Research, 2*:1, pp. 7-26, 1992.

Roberto, K. A., Equity in Friendships, in *Older Adult Friendships*, R. G. Adams and R. Blieszner (eds.), Sage Publications, Inc., Newbury Park, California, pp. 147-165, 1989.

Roberto, K. and J. Scott, Equity Considerations in Friendships of Older Adults, *Journal of Gerontology, 41*, pp. 241-247, 1986.

Robinson, B. and M. Thurnher, Taking Care of Aged Parents, *The Gerontologist, 19*, pp. 586-593, 1979.

Rodman, H., *Lower Class Families: The Culture of Poverty in Negro Trinidad*, Oxford University Press, New York, 1971.

Rook, K. S., Reciprocity of Social Exchange and Social Satisfaction Among Older Women, *Journal of Personality and Social Psychology, 62*, pp. 145-154, 1987.

Rook, K. S., Strains in Older Adults' Friendships, in *Older Adult Friendships*, R. G. Adams and R. Blieszner (eds.), Sage Publications, Inc., Newbury Park, California, pp. 166-196, 1989.

Rosel, N., The Hub of a Wheel: A Neighborhood Support Network, *International Journal of Aging and Human Development, 16*, pp. 193-200, 1983.

Rosenberg, M., *Conceiving the Self*, Basic Books, New York, 1979.

Rosenbloom, C. A. and F. J. Whittington, The Effects of Bereavement on Eating Behaviors and Nutrient Intakes in Elderly Widowed Persons, *Journal of Gerontology: Social Sciences, 48*:4, pp. S223-S229, 1993.

Rosow, I., *Social Integration of the Aged*, The Free Press, New York, 1967.

Rosow, I., *Socialization to Old Age*, University of California Press, Berkeley, California, 1974.

Ross, J. K., *Old People, New Lives: Community Creation in A Retirement Residence*, University of Chicago Press, Chicago, 1977.

Rothman, J., A Model of Case Management: Toward Empirically Based Practice, *Social Work, 36*, pp. 520-527, 1991.

Rubinstein, R. L., B. B. Alexander, M. Goodman, and M. Luborsky, Key Relationships of Never Married, Childless Older Women: A Cultural Analysis, *Journal of Gerontology: Social Sciences, 46*:5, pp. S270-S277, 1991.

Rubinstein, R. L., J. C. Kilbride, and S. Nagy, *Elders Living Alone*, Aldine de Gruyter, New York, 1992.

Sabatino, C. P., Client Rights Regulations and the Autonomy of Home-Care Consumers, *Generations, XIV*:Supplement, pp. 21-24, 1990.

Sahlins, M., On the Sociology of Primitive Exchange, in *The Relevance of Models for Social Anthropology*, M. Banton (ed.), Praeger, New York, 1965.

Savishinsky, J., *The Ends of Time: Life and Work in a Nursing Home*, Bergin and Garvey, New York, 1991.

Schulz, R. and G. M. Williamson, Psychosocial and Behavioral Dimensions of Physical Frailty, *Journal of Gerontology, 48*:Supplement, pp. 39-43, 1993.

Scott, J. P., Siblings and Other Kin, in *Family Relations in Later Life*, T. H. Brubaker (ed.), Sage Publications, Inc., Beverly Hills, California, 1983.

Seelbach, W., Filial Responsibility Among Aged Parents: A Racial Comparison, *Journal of Minority Aging, 5*, pp. 286-292, 1980.

Shanas, E., Social Myth as Hypothesis: The Case of Family Relations of Old People, *The Gerontologist, 19*, pp. 3-9, 1979.

Shanas, E., The Family as a Social Support System in Old Age, *The Gerontologist, 19*, pp. 64-69, 1979.

Shanas, E., Older People and Their Families: The New Pioneers, *Journal of Marriage and the Family, 42*, pp. 9-15, 1980.

Sheehan, S., *Kate Quinton's Days*, New American Library, New York, 1984.

Sherman, S., Mutual Assistance and Support in Retirement Housing, *Journal of Gerontology, 30*, pp. 479-483, 1975.

Sherwood, S. and J. Morris, The Pennsylvania Domiciliary Care Experiment: 1. Impact on Quality of Life, *American Journal of Public Health, 73*, pp. 646-653, 1983.

Shield, R., *Uneasy Endings: Daily Life in an American Nursing Home*, Cornell University Press, Ithaca, New York, 1988.

Smithers, J., *Determined Survivors: Community Life Among the Urban Elderly*, Rutgers University Press, New Brunswick, New Jersey, 1985.

Sokolovsky, J. and C. Cohen, Being Old in the Inner City: Support Systems of the SRO Aged, in *Aging in Culture and Society: Comparative Viewpoints and Strategies*, C. Fry (ed.), J. F. Bergin, Brooklyn, pp. 163-181, 1980.

Sorgen, L., The Development of a Home Care Quality Assurance Program in Alberta, *Home Health Care Services Quarterly*, 7:1, pp. 13-28, 1986.

Stack, C., *All Our Kin*, Harper and Row, New York, 1974.

Starrett, R. A., Home Health Care: The Elderly's Perception, *Home Health Care Services Quarterly*, 7:1, pp. 69-79, 1986.

Stoller, E., Parental Caregiving by Adult Children, *Journal of Marriage and the Family, 45*, pp. 851-858, 1983.

Stoller, E., Exchange Patterns in the Informal Networks of the Elderly: The Impact on Morale, *Journal of Marriage and the Family, 47*, pp. 851-857, 1985.

Stoller, E., Long-term Care Planning by Informal Helpers: Likelihood of Shared Households and Institutional Placement, *Journal of Applied Gerontology, 7*, pp. 5-20, 1988.

Stoller, E. P. and S. J. Cutler, Predictors of Use of Paid Help Among Older People Living in the Community, *The Gerontologist, 33*:1, pp. 31-40, 1993.

Stoller, E. and L. Earl, Help with Activities of Everyday Life: Sources of Support for the Non-institutionalized Elderly, *The Gerontologist, 23*, pp. 64-69, 1983.

Stoller, E. P. and K. L. Pugliesi, Size and Effectiveness of Informal Helping Networks: A Panel Study of Older People in the Community, *Journal of Health and Social Behavior, 32*:2, pp. 180-191, 1991.

Stone, R., G. L. Cafferata, and J. Sangl, Caregivers of the Frail Elderly: A National Profile, *The Gerontologist, 27*:5, pp. 616-626, 1987.

Stryker, S. and R. Serpe, Commitment, Identity Salience and Role Behavior: Theory and Research Example, in *Personality, Roles, and Social Behavior*, W. Ickes and E. S. Knowles (eds.), Springer-Verlag, New York, pp. 199-218, 1982.

Surpin, R. and F. Grumm, Building the Home Care Triangle: Clients and Families, Paraprofessionals and Agencies, *Caring*, pp. 6-15, 1990.

Sussman, M. B., The Family Life of Old People, in *Handbook of Aging and the Social Sciences*, R. H. Binstock and E. Shanas (eds.), Van Nostrand Reinhold, New York, pp. 218-243, 1976.

Tammivaara, J. and D. S. Enright, On Eliciting Information: Dialogues with Child Informants, *Anthropology and Education Quarterly, 17*, pp. 218-238, 1986.

Thomas, D., D. Franks, and J. Calonico, Role-taking and Power in Social Psychology, *American Sociological Review, 37*, pp. 128-137, 1972.

Thornton, R. and P. Nardi, The Dynamics of Role Acquisition, *American Journal of Sociology, 80*, pp. 870-883, 1975.

Treas, J., Family Support Systems for the Aged, *The Gerontologist, 17*, pp. 486-491, 1977.

Turner, R., Role Taking: Process Versus Conformity, in *Human Behavior and Social Process*, A. Rose (ed.), Houghton Mifflin, Boston, 1962.

Turner, R. H., Unanswered Questions in the Convergence between Structuralist and Interactionist, in *Micro-Theory*, H. J. Helle and S. N. Eisenstadt (eds.), Vol. 2, Sage Publications, Inc., London, 1985.

Twaddle, A. and R. Hessler, *A Sociology of Health* (2nd Edition), C. V. Mosby, St. Louis, 1987.

U.S. General Accounting Office, *Long-Term Care: Status of Quality Assurance and Measurement in Home and Community-Based Services*, Report to the Chairman, Committee on Finance, U.S. Senate, Washington, D.C., March 1994.

U.S. House of Representatives Select Committee on Aging, Long-Term Care and Personal Impoverishment: Seven in Eleven Elderly Living Alone Are at Risk, U.S. Congress, October 1987.

Van Nostrand, J., *Health Data on Older Americans*, United States Public Health Service, Series 3, No. 27, 1993.

Vicusi, W. K., An Assessment of Aid to the Elderly: Incentive Effects and the Elderly's Role in Society, in *Aging, Stability, and Family Change*, J. March (ed.), Academic Press, New York, 1981.

Walls, C. T. and S. H. Zarit, Informal Support from Black Churches and the Well-Being of Elderly Blacks, *The Gerontologist, 31*:4, pp. 490-495, 1991.

Wallston, K. and B. S. Wallston, Health Locus of Control Studies, in *Research with the Locus of Control Concept*, H. Lefcourt (ed.), Vol. 1, Academic Press, New York, pp. 189-243, 1981.

Wan, T. and W. Weissert, Social Support Networks, Patient Status and Institutionalization, *Research on Aging, 3*, pp. 240-256, 1981.

Wan, T., W. Weissert, and R. Livieratos, Geriatric Daycare and Homemaker Services: An Experimental Study, *Journal of Gerontology, 35*, pp. 256-274, 1980.

Weber, M., *From Max Weber: Essays in Sociology*, H. Gerth and C. W. Mills (eds. and trans.), Oxford University Press, New York, 1958.

Weinstein, E., The Development of Interpersonal Competence, in *Handbook of Socialization Theory and Research*, D. Goslin (ed.), Rand McNally, Chicago, 1969.

Weiss, H., Quality of Care: Bringing it into the Community, *Contemporary LTC*, pp. 24-26, 1987.

Weissert, W., Seven Reasons Why it is so Difficult to Make Community-based Long-term Care Cost-effective, *Health Services Research, 20*, pp. 20-24, 1985.

Weissert, W., C. Cready, and J. Pawelak, The Past and Future of Community-based Long-term Care, *The Milbank Quarterly, 66*, pp. 309-388, 1988.

Wellin, E. and E. Boyer, Adjustments of Black and White Elderly to the Same Adaptive Niche, *Anthropological Quarterly, 52*, pp. 39-46, 1979.

Wenger, G. C., Dependence, Interdependency, and Reciprocity After 80, *Journal of Aging Studies, 1*, pp. 355-377, 1987.

Wenger, G. C., Personal Care: Variations in Network Type, Style and Capacity, in *The Home Care Experience*, J. F. Gubrium and A. Sankar (eds.), Sage Publications, Inc., Newbury Park, California, pp. 145-172, 1990.

Wentowski, G. J., Reciprocity and the Coping Strategies of Older People: Cultural Dimensions of Network Building, *The Gerontologist, 21*, pp. 600-609, 1981.

White-Means, S. I., Informal Home Care for Frail Black Elderly, *Journal of Applied Gerontology, 12*:1, pp. 13-33, 1993.

Whittington, F. J., Drugs, Aging, and Social Policy, in *Drugs and the Elderly: Social and Pharmacological Issues*, D. M. Petersen, F. J. Whittington, and B. P. Payne (eds.), Charles C. Thomas, Publisher, Springfield, Illinois, 1979.

Whittington, F. J., Misuse of Legal Drugs and Compliance with Prescription Directions, in *Drugs and the Elderly Adult*, M. D. Glantz, D. M. Petersen, and F. J. Whittington (eds.), U.S. Department of Health and Human Services, Washington, D.C., pp. 63-69, 1983.

Whyte, W. H., *Street Corner Society*, University of Chicago Press, Chicago, 1955.

Wister, A. V., Environmental Adaptation by Persons in Their Later Life, *Research on Aging, 11*:3, pp. 267-291, 1989.

Yee, B. W. K. and G. D. Weaver, Ethnic Minorities and Health Promotion: Developing a "Culturally Competent Agenda," *Generations, XVIII*:1, pp. 39-44, 1994.

# Author Index

Abel, E. K., 106, 148
Abeles, R. P., 124
Adams, R. G., 89, 124, 149, 256
Administration on Aging, 13
Agency for Health Care Policy and Research, 12
Alexander, B. B., 52, 107
Allan, G. A., 89, 124
Allen, K. R., 107, 118, 124, 148
Altholz, J. A., 231, 256
American Association of Retired Persons, 12
American Health Care Association, 12
Antonucci, T. C., 89
Applebaum, R., 13, 187
Aschenbrenner, J., 14, 147

Banton, M., 146
Barer, B. M., 106, 122, 125, 147, 204
Barker, J. C., 106, 135, 146
Barry, C., 105
Berg, S., 88, 187
Berk, M. L., 11
Bernard, S., 52
Berwick, D., 186, 187
Besdine, R. W., 124
Binstock, R. H., 11, 107, 147
Blieszner, R., 89, 124, 149, 256
Bloom, S. W., 210, 231
Bottomore, T., 14
Boyer, E., 89
Branch, L. G., 105

Braun, K. L., 13, 187
Brody, E., 12, 148
Brody, S. J., 105
Brown, R., 13, 187
Brubaker, T. H., 106

Cafferata, G. L., 148
Calonico, J., 214, 231
Cantor, M., 12, 72, 104, 105, 132, 146, 147, 168, 241, 245
Capitman, J., 13, 187
Carcagno, G., 13, 187
Carlsson-Agren, M., 75, 88, 170, 187
Carson, W., 13, 187
Catalano, D. J., 105, 146, 148
Challis, D., 13
Chappell, N. L., 236, 255
Chatters, L. M., 105
Chichin, E., 168, 241, 245
Chin-Sang, V., 107, 118, 124, 148
Choi, N. G., 12
Christianson, J., 13, 187
Chubon, S. J., 61, 72
Cleary, P. D., 124
Cohen, C., 88, 148
Colligen, F., 13, 187
Collopy, B. J., 110, 124
Corbin, J. M., 230, 231
Corder, L. S., 11
Cowan, C. A., 12
Cready, C., 13
Crohan, S. E., 89
Crossman, L., 105

# Subject Index

# Author Biographies

MARY M. BALL received her M.S. in sociology from Emory University and her Ph.D. in sociology from Georgia State University. Her research includes qualitative studies of reciprocal exchange among welfare mothers, the role of informal caregiving in the black community, and the long-term care experiences of African American elders.

Dr. Ball currently works with the Georgia Long-Term Care Ombudsman Program. Most recently she was Director of Programs for Older Adults at Emmaus House, a community center located in a low-income area of Atlanta where she had worked as a volunteer for twenty years.

FRANK J. WHITTINGTON is Professor of Sociology at Georgia State University in Atlanta and a Research Health Scientist at the Atlanta VA Rehabilitation Research and Development Center on Aging. During 1991-93, he worked at the National Institute on Aging as Senior Research Policy Advisor for the Task Force on Aging Research, a congressionally-mandated federal body that developed policy recommendations on aging research.

Dr. Whittington received his Ph.D. from Duke University where he was a Research Training Program Fellow in the Center for the Study of Aging and Human Development. He is a Fellow of the Gerontological Society of America, and his publications include four books and over thirty articles and chapters on long-term care and health behavior of older people, particularly the use and misuse of medications. His current research focuses on the physical and chemical restraint of nursing home residents.